RAINBOW

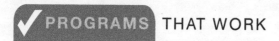 **PROGRAMS** THAT WORK

RAINBOW

A Child- and Family-Focused Cognitive-Behavioral Treatment
for Pediatric Bipolar Disorder

CLINICIAN GUIDE

AMY E. WEST
SALLY M. WEINSTEIN
MANI N. PAVULURI

OXFORD
UNIVERSITY PRESS

OXFORD
UNIVERSITY PRESS

Oxford University Press is a department of the University of Oxford. It furthers
the University's objective of excellence in research, scholarship, and education
by publishing worldwide. Oxford is a registered trade mark of Oxford University
Press in the UK and certain other countries.

Published in the United States of America by Oxford University Press
198 Madison Avenue, New York, NY 10016, United States of America.

Library of Congress Cataloging-in-Publication Data
Names: West, Amy E., author. | Weinstein, Sally M., author. | Pavuluri, Mani N., author.
Title: Rainbow : a child- and family-focused cognitive-behavioral treatment for pediatric
bipolar disorder : clinician guide / Amy E. West, Sally M. Weinstein, Mani N. Pavuluri.
Description: Oxford ; New York : Oxford University Press, [2018] | Series: Programs that work series
Identifiers: LCCN 2017022823 (print) | LCCN 2017030965 (ebook) | ISBN 9780190609146 (updf) |
ISBN 9780190671662 (epub) | ISBN 9780190609139 (paperback)
Subjects: LCSH: Manic-depressive illness in children—Treatment. | Cognitive therapy. |
Parent and child.
Classification: LCC RJ506.D4 (ebook) | LCC RJ506.D4 W47 2018 (print) |
DDC 618.9289/5—dc23
LC record available at https://lccn.loc.gov/2017022823

9 8 7 6 5 4 3 2 1

Printed by WebCom, Inc., Canada

Stunning developments in healthcare have taken place over the last several years, but many of our widely accepted interventions and strategies in mental health and behavioral medicine have been brought into question by research evidence as not only lacking benefit, but perhaps, inducing harm (Barlow, 2010). Other strategies have been proven effective using the best current standards of evidence, resulting in broad-based recommendations to make these practices more available to the public (McHugh & Barlow, 2012). Several recent developments are behind this revolution. First, we have arrived at a much deeper understanding of pathology, both psychological and physical, which has led to the development of new, more precisely targeted interventions. Second, our research methodologies have improved substantially, such that we have reduced threats to internal and external validity, making the outcomes more directly applicable to clinical situations. Third, governments around the world and healthcare systems and policymakers have decided that the quality of care should improve, that it should be evidence based, and that it is in the public's interest to ensure that this happens (Barlow, 2004; Institute of Medicine, 2001, 2015; Weisz & Kazdin, 2017).

Of course, the major stumbling block for clinicians everywhere is the accessibility of newly developed evidence-based psychological interventions. Workshops and books can go only so far in acquainting responsible and conscientious practitioners with the latest behavioral healthcare practices and their applicability to individual patients. This new series, Programs *ThatWork*™, is devoted to communicating these exciting new interventions to clinicians on the frontlines of practice.

The manuals and workbooks in this series contain step-by-step detailed procedures for assessing and treating specific problems and diagnoses. But this series also goes beyond the books and manuals by providing ancillary materials that will approximate the supervisory process in assisting practitioners in the implementation of these procedures in their practice.

In our emerging healthcare system, the growing consensus is that evidence-based practice offers the most responsible course of action for the mental health professional. All behavioral healthcare clinicians deeply desire to provide the best possible care for their patients. In this series, our aim is to close the dissemination and information gap and make that possible.

This Clinician Guide presents a structured, 12-session program called Child- and Family-Focused Cognitive-Behavioral Therapy (CFF-CBT, or *RAINBOW* therapy) for children aged 7–13 with pediatric bipolar disorder (PBD) and their families. PBD is associated with chronic, severe symptoms that result in emotional, behavioral, and social difficulties and a range of impairments for affected youth. To date, there are few evidence-based psychosocial treatments for PBD, and the developmentally specific approach of RAINBOW for this age group is a welcome addition. The program has been shown to significantly improve mood symptoms and overall functioning in children while also addressing the needs of parents, so therapy includes intensive work for both. This Guide includes clear instructions for each session as well as all necessary handouts, worksheets, and activities to be completed during therapy.

Anne Marie Albano, Editor-in-Chief
David H. Barlow, Editor-in-Chief
Programs *ThatWork*

References

Barlow, D.H. (2004). Psychological treatments. *American Psychologist, 59*, 869–878.

Barlow, D.H. (2010). Negative effects from psychological treatments: A perspective. *American Psychologist, 65(2)*, 13–20.

Institute of Medicine. (2001). *Crossing the quality chasm: A new health system for the 21st century.* Washington, DC: National Academy Press.

Institute of Medicine. (2015). *Psychosocial interventions for mental and substance use disorders: a framework for establishing evidence-based standards.* Washington, DC: National Academy Press

McHugh, R.K., & Barlow, D.H. (2012). *Dissemination and implementation of evidence-based psychological interventions.* Oxford: Oxford University Press.

Weisz, J. R., & Kazdin, A. E. (2017). *Evidence-based Psychotherapies for Children and Adolescents* (3rd ed.). Guilford.

Accessing Program *ThatWork* Forms and Worksheets Online

Forms and worksheets from books in the PTW Series are made available digitally shortly following print publication. You may download, print, save, and digitally complete them as PDFs. To access the forms and worksheets, please visit http://www.oup.com/us/ttw.

Acknowledgments

The authors would like to thank Julie Carbray, Ph.D., and Jodi Heidenreich, L.C.S.W., for their role in the development and early implementation of CFF-CBT/RAINBOW. The authors would also like to thank the many graduate students that served as CFF-CBT/RAINBOW therapists and provided valuable feedback and input during treatment development and refinement. Finally, the authors would like to express their gratitude for all of the children and families who participated in CFF-CBT/RAINBOW and provided essential information pertinent to implementing the treatment model.

Contents

RAINBOW

Introduction

Pediatric bipolar disorder (PBD) is characterized by extreme mood dysregulation and a complex constellation of symptoms that contribute to significant impairment in psychosocial functioning. Relative to the adult presentation of bipolar disorder, the pediatric presentation is characterized by more rapid cycling, mixed mood episodes, and psychiatric comorbidity. Over time, these impairments and the chronic and severe symptoms associated with pediatric bipolar disorder accumulate, resulting in significant emotional, behavioral, and social difficulties for these youth. Psychosocial impairment in pediatric bipolar disorder is evidenced by academic difficulties and behavioral issues at school; significant social impairment, including few or no relationships with peers, and poor social skills; and conflict and tension within the family unit, including disruptions in sibling and parent relationships (West & Weinstein, 2011). Thus, adjunctive psychosocial treatments are imperative to address the range of functional impairments associated with pediatric bipolar disorder that are not addressed by pharmacological treatment alone.

To date, a limited number of psychosocial treatments have been developed and tested for pediatric bipolar disorder. The efficacy of two other psychosocial treatments has been rigorously tested in randomized controlled trials (RCTs): multi-family psychoeducation group psychotherapy (MF-PEP) for children aged 8–12 with a mood disorder (e.g., bipolar disorder, dysthymic disorder, or major depressive disorder) (Fristad, Verducci, Walters, & Young, 2009), and family-focused treatment adapted for adolescents (FFT-A) aged 13–18 years with bipolar disorder (Miklowitz et al., 2008). MF-PEP demonstrated reductions in mood symptom severity (Fristad et al., 2009), and FFT demonstrated significant reductions in depression relapse (Miklowitz et al., 2008). Two additional treatments—dialectical behavior therapy (Goldstein et al., 2015) and interpersonal and social rhythm therapy (Hlastala, Kotler, McClellan, & McCauley, 2010)—have been adapted for adolescents with bipolar disorder and have undergone preliminary testing in pilot trials.

Child- and Family-Focused Cognitive-Behavioral Therapy (CFF-CBT, or RAINBOW therapy) was developed as an adjunctive psychosocial intervention to meet the developmental needs of children 7–13 with bipolar spectrum disorders, and their families (Pavuluri et al., 2004; West, Henry, & Pavuluri, 2007; West et al., 2009; West & Pavuluri, 2009; West et al., 2014). We believe that CFF-CBT comprises four innovative aspects in the treatment of pediatric bipolar disorder, in that it:

(1) Is designed to be developmentally specific to children aged 7–13;
(2) Is driven by the distinct needs of these children with bipolar disorder and their families (e.g., affect modulation);
(3) Involves intensive work with parents parallel to the work with children in order to directly address parents' own therapeutic needs, as well as helping them develop an effective parenting style for their child with bipolar disorder; and
(4) Integrates psychoeducation, cognitive-behavioral therapy, and interpersonal therapy techniques, tailored to the unique needs of these children.

Diverse therapeutic techniques are employed across multiple domains, including individual, peer, family, and school, to address the impact of pediatric bipolar disorder in the child's broader psychosocial context. We refer to all caregivers as "parents" throughout the manual, although occasionally we refer to "caregivers." Our intention is to attribute the role of parent to any caregiver who takes on the role of caring for the child.

Empirical Foundation for CFF-CBT

As shown in Figure 1, the psychotherapeutic methods used in CFF-CBT are driven by three areas of research evidence:

(1) Affective circuitry brain dysfunction in pediatric bipolar disorder (e.g., poor problem solving during affective stimulation due to underactivity in dorsolateral prefrontal cortex);
(2) Developmentally specific symptoms of pediatric bipolar disorder (e.g., rapid cycling, mixed mood states, comorbid disorders); and

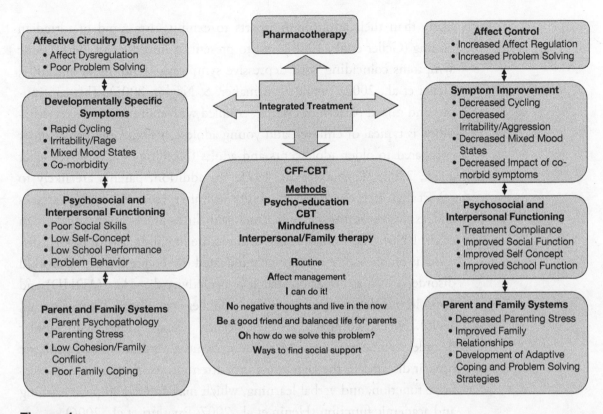

Figure 1

Conceptual Model for CFF-CBT/RAINBOW.

(3) The impact of pediatric bipolar disorder on psychosocial and interpersonal functioning.

First, studies of biological dysfunction in pediatric bipolar disorder implicate the brain structures involved in affective circuitry, including the dorsolateral prefrontal cortex (DLPFC), ventrolateral prefrontal cortex (VLPFC), superior temporal and visual cortices, and amygdala (Garrett et al., 2012; Mayberg, 1997; Passarotti & Pavuluri, 2011; Rich et al., 2011; Yurgelun-Todd et al., 2000). The DLPFC is implicated in problem-solving, while the VLPFC and amygdala work in concert to regulate affective responses (Mayberg, 1997). Functional neuroimaging studies have demonstrated reduced activation in the DLPFC and VLPFC, possibly contributing to problem-solving difficulties during excessive emotional reactivity and increased activation of the amygdala (Garrett et al., 2012; Mayberg, 1997; Passarotti & Pavuluri, 2011; Rich et al., 2011; Yurgelun-Todd et al., 2000).

Second, children with bipolar disorder evidence many unique symptom patterns that require tailored intervention. For example, they are more likely than their adult counterparts to exhibit ultra-rapid or ultradian cycling (Geller et al., 1998), and to present in mixed states, with manic symptoms coinciding with depressive symptoms (Findling et al., 2001; Geller et al., 2002; Pavuluri, Birmaher, & Naylor, 2005). This continuous and mixed pattern of cycling, coupled with more pronounced irritability, is typical of children and young adolescents with bipolar disorder compared to older adolescents and adults (Findling et al., 2001; Geller et al., 2002; Wozniak et al., 1995). In addition, parents are likely to report that their children's irritability will often escalate into rage attacks and explosive outbursts, sometimes with little provocation (Biederman et al., 1996). The complex symptom picture in children with bipolar disorder is often made even more complicated by the presence of comorbid disorders, such as attention-deficit hyperactivity disorders (ADHD) and oppositional defiant disorder (ODD) (Geller et al., 2002; Wozniak et al., 1995). Finally, compared to their healthy peers, children with bipolar disorder demonstrate trait-level neurocognitive dysfunction in pediatric bipolar disorder in the key domains of attention, working memory, executive function, and verbal learning, which may severely impede learning and academic function (Henin et al., 2007; Pavuluri et al., 2006).

Third, due to the rapid mood changes and recalcitrant nature of the disorder—from irritable, excitable, impulsive, intrusive, and loud, to sullen, withdrawn, and weepy—these children often have significant interpersonal problems with peers and family members (Geller et al., 2002). Peer rejection and family conflict may erode the child's sense of self and contribute to feelings of worthlessness (Pavuluri et al., 2004). Conflict and expressed emotion often result from the exhaustion and strain endured by parents (Miklowitz et al., 2004). Specifically, compared to families unaffected by pediatric bipolar disorder, family functioning is often characterized by strained relationships (Geller et al., 2000; Wilens et al., 2003), lower cohesion, and increased conflict (Goldstein, Miklowitz, & Mullen, 2006; Rucklidge, 2006; Schenkel, West, Harral, Patel, & Pavuluri, 2008); family stress and dysfunction have been shown to increase with symptom levels (Keenan-Miller, Peris, Axelson, Kowatch, & Miklowitz, 2012; Kim, Miklowitz, Biuckians, & Mullen, 2007).

Organization and Essential Components of CFF-CBT

The core concepts and initial CFF-CBT curricula were developed based on the scientific understanding of affective circuitry, developmentally specific symptoms, and psychosocial and interpersonal functioning in pediatric bipolar disorder. CFF-CBT is a 12-session protocol-driven treatment program meant to be delivered weekly over the course of three months (see Table 1). Each session is 60–90 minutes. Many of the sessions are for the parent and child together, but some are individual sessions for the parent or the child. CFF-CBT has also been adapted to a group format, which consists of parallel parent and child groups that run for 1½ hours each week for 12 weeks. Although CFF-CBT was tested based on the established content and sequence of the manual, and thus adherence to the protocol is most predictive of outcomes, the treatment protocol may be implemented in a flexible manner to best meet the family's needs or to work within timing constraints, as long as the essential ingredients are included. For example, 90-minute parent sessions may be shortened by adapting the content to the most salient aspects for the parent. The acronym "RAINBOW" was formed to help parents and children remember the key components of CFF-CBT; these essential ingredients are described in more detail in the following sections.

R: Routine

The goal of the Routine component is to increase affect regulation and decrease symptom exacerbation by establishing a predictable, simplified routine to reduce excessive reactivity and tense negotiations in response to changes in the child's schedule. Parents are encouraged to establish routines around sleep, diet, medication, and transitions. Parents are also urged to integrate soothing and pleasurable activities into their own and their child's routine.

A: Affect Regulation

The goal of the Affect Regulation component is to provide psychoeducation about symptoms of pediatric bipolar disorder and neurochemical underpinnings, teach behavioral management and coping strategies, and provide affective education to the children. Parents are educated about the biological basis of their child's illness and the nature of bipolar symptoms. Parents are instructed in various behavioral management techniques, borrowed from Barkley (1987) and Greene (2001), to establish appropriate systems for negotiation and creating consistent consequences. Children are educated about recognizing and responding to affective states and consistently self-monitoring moods; they are given a system to monitor their moods several times throughout each day.

I: I Can Do It!

The goal of the I Can Do It component is to increase parents' and children's beliefs in their ability to cope with the disorder and to problem-solve issues. CFF-CBT employs techniques designed to increase a sense of self-efficacy in children and parents, including having children and parents generate a list of positive self-statements, encouraging parents to focus on their child's positive qualities, and helping parents give consistent positive reinforcement for good behavior. Parents are encouraged to approach interactions with their children using a mixture of quiet confidence, firm limit-setting, calming tones, empathy, and a focus on positive reframing, which we believe to be an effective combination for children who are highly sensitive to criticism and whose negative mood states are easily triggered. This style of interaction is likely to be more effective than shouting, threatening, and/or swift punishment in regulating the child's response, and it instills a sense of confidence in both the child and parent that the particular situation will be resolved positively.

N: No Negative Thoughts and Live in the Now!

The goals of the No Negative Thoughts, Live in the Now component are twofold. The first goal is to decrease negative thinking and thought distortions associated with depression. Children and families are taught how to differentiate between helpful and unhelpful thoughts and to reframe unhelpful thoughts into helpful ones that increase their sense of hope, beliefs in efficacy around coping, and ability to solve problems. The second goal of this component is to encourage children and parents to focus on the present moment and to avoid becoming overwhelmed by thoughts of what might happen in the future. Based on evidence from the emerging literature on the use of mindfulness techniques in cognitive-behavioral therapy for depression (Segal, Williams, & Teasdale, 2002), children and parents are encouraged to focus on coping in the present moment, rather than dwelling on past failures or anticipating future failures. Mindfulness techniques, such as the use of positive mantras, are incorporated.

B: Be a Good Friend and Balanced Lifestyle for Parents

The first goal of the Be a Good Friend, Balanced Lifestyle for Parents component is to improve social functioning in children. Children with bipolar disorder often have significant difficulties in peer relationships; a major goal of this component is to help children establish and maintain friendships. Children are taught the skills necessary to be a good friend and are provided opportunities within the therapy session to practice the skills. Parents are also encouraged to seek opportunities for children to practice newly developed skills and develop friendships (such as sleepovers, play dates, and supervised group activities). The second goal is to increase parents' sense of well-being and their ability to cope by achieving a balanced lifestyle. Parents of children with bipolar disorder often suffer from physical and emotional exhaustion, frustration, guilt, and feelings of isolation (Fristad & Goldberg-Arnold, 2003). Therefore, we encourage parents to develop a more balanced lifestyle that involves finding ways to rest, replenish their energy, and enjoy life. As an initial strategy related to this goal, parents draw a pie diagram that depicts the amount of time they invest in "recharging their own batteries" versus being a spouse, worker, or parent. Then, together, the therapist and the parents discuss how to "carve the pie" so that parents strike a healthier balance between the demands of caring for a child with bipolar disorder and taking care of themselves.

O: Oh, How Can We Solve the Problem?

The goal of Oh, How Can We Solve the Problem component is to engage parents and children in a collaborative and effective problem-solving process. Parents are encouraged to view their children as partners in the problem-solving process and to explain the pros and cons of potential solutions in an empathic way. Parents and children are encouraged to try creative ways to approach problem-solving in order to minimize reactivity and the exacerbation of negative emotion.

W: Ways to Get Support

The goal of the Ways to Get Support component is to increase social support. Isolation, shame, and lack of access may prevent parents of children with bipolar disorder from finding friends or family members who can provide respite and support. Therefore, the techniques used in this component emphasize the identification and active seeking-out of people who can help the child and the parents through difficult situations. School advocacy is also a part of this component. Teachers may be provided with a portfolio of CFF-CBT materials, including information about the diagnosis and about ways in which the disorder may interfere with a child's performance in school. Parents are encouraged to engage the child's individual therapist or school counselor in further advocating for the child's needs at school.

Session Topics

Table 1 summarizes information about the 12 individual treatment sessions, including who is present in each session, the topics covered, and the required materials.

Table 1 Summary of 12 Treatment Sessions

Session	Participants	Topics Covered	Required Materials
1	Child and parents together	▪ Orientation to treatment/goal-setting ▪ Engagement and relationship-building	Handouts #1–6
2	Child and parents together	▪ Psychoeducation about PBD ▪ Mood charting	Handouts #7–10; prize basket
3	Parents only	▪ Affect regulation ▪ Establishing routines; identifying difficult feelings; anger management	Handouts #11–12
4	Child only	▪ Affect-regulation skills ▪ Labeling emotions; recognizing difficult feelings; triggers	Handouts #9 and #13–18; prize basket
5	Child only	▪ Coping skills ▪ Problem solving; positive thinking	Handouts #9 and #19–23, prize basket
6	Parents only	▪ Positive thinking; mantras; reframing negative thoughts; mindfulness	Handouts #24–27
7	Child only	▪ Communication skills and interpersonal problem solving	Handouts #9 and #28–32; prize basket
8	Parents only	▪ Promoting social competence; behavior management; balanced life	Handouts #17 and #33–34, pen
9	Parents, child, siblings	▪ Family coping and problem solving	Handout #35; prize basket
10	Child and parents together	▪ Social support	Handouts #36–37; markers, pencils, or crayons
11	Child and parents together	▪ Reflection on RAINBOW experience and review	RAINBOW binder; 3 copies of Handout #1; Handout #13; Handout #38; construction paper
12	Child and parents together	▪ Celebration; follow-up plan	None

The preliminary open trial of CFF-CBT (Pavuluri et al., 2004) was conducted to assess its feasibility, child adherence to the treatment (including dropouts), therapist adherence to the treatment protocol, and parent satisfaction with their treatment experience. In addition, outcome measures were administered to explore the effect of the treatment on symptom severity and overall functioning. Thirty-four children and young adolescents were assessed for bipolar symptoms and global functioning before and after treatment. Results indicated that the CFF-CBT intervention was feasible to deliver, and that children were very satisfied with their experience. In addition, preliminary evidence demonstrated a reduction in symptoms of attention problems, aggression, mania, psychosis, depression, and sleep disturbance, and increased global functioning after the intervention.

Despite these encouraging initial gains, our clinical experience has taught us that these improvements are unlikely to be sustained without continued maintenance treatment. Therefore, we conducted a study of a maintenance model of CFF-CBT, comprising psychosocial booster sessions and optimized pharmacotherapy (West et al., 2007). The 34 patients who underwent the initial 12-session treatment were followed over a three-year period and assessed for symptom experience and global functioning at years 1, 2, and 3 during the maintenance phase. During these three years, maintenance treatment consisted of ongoing medication management with psychosocial booster sessions using the CFF-CBT ingredients. Results indicated that the children were able to maintain initial positive effects of the treatment over the three-year follow-up period with continued booster treatment. These findings suggest that maintenance treatment models may help facilitate the long-term management of symptoms and represent an important step in addressing the low recovery and high relapse rates associated with pediatric bipolar disorder.

A randomized clinical trial of CFF-CBT (West et al., 2014) was recently completed to assess the efficacy of CFF-CBT in reducing acute mood symptoms and improving global psychosocial functioning among youth with bipolar disorder. Sixty-nine youth with a bipolar spectrum diagnosis, and their families, were randomly assigned to CFF-CBT or psychotherapy treatment as usual (TAU). Both groups received 12 weekly treatment sessions during the acute phase of treatment, and six monthly booster sessions. Youth and their parents were assessed on measures of psychosocial functioning at baseline; 4, 8, and 12 weeks (post-treatment); and again at 39 weeks (six-month follow-up). Results indicated that youth in CFF-CBT experienced a greater reduction in parent-reported mania symptoms at post-treatment, and in depression symptoms at post-treatment and follow-up, relative to youth in TAU. At post-treatment, global psychosocial functioning did not differ between groups, but youth in CFF-CBT had higher global functioning at follow-up relative to youth in TAU. In addition, CFF-CBT resulted in greater levels of engagement among families, indicated by better attendance, fewer dropouts, and greater satisfaction with treatment, compared to TAU. Thus, these results suggest that CFF-CBT may be particularly effective at improving outcomes among youth with pediatric bipolar disorder. Moreover, results indicated that CFF-CBT was relatively immune to the presence of several factors that could potentially complicate treatment: Children of parents with higher depressive symptoms showed greater response to CFF-CBT versus TAU in terms of their own depression symptoms and, marginally, overall psychiatric severity. Similarly, we saw that children from low-income families showed greater response to CFF-CBT relative to TAU (Weinstein et al., 2015).

Finally, CFF-CBT has also been adapted to a group format, comprising 12 weeks of parallel parent and child groups. The group treatment is manual-based and delivers the same content as is delivered in the individual-treatment format. However, parent support and skill building are enhanced through the interchange that occurs when multiple parents are present in a single group session. A preliminary open trial of the CFF-CBT group treatment was completed to test its feasibility. Results indicated that the group adaptation was feasible to deliver and resulted in a significant increase in parents' report of their child's coping skills, a decrease in parenting stress, an increase in parents' knowledge and self-efficacy in coping with the disorder, and a decrease in parent-reported symptoms of mania after treatment (West et al., 2009).

References

Barkley, R. A. (1987). *Defiant Children: A Clinician's Manual for Parent Training*. New York: Guilford Press.

Biederman, J., Faraone, S., Milberger, S., Guite, J., Mick, E., Chen, L., . . . Moore, P. (1996). A prospective 4-year follow-up study of attention-deficit hyperactivity and related disorders. *Archives of General Psychiatry, 53*(5), 437–446.

Findling, R. L., Gracious, B. L., McNamara, N. K., Youngstrom, E. A., Demeter, C. A., Branicky, L. A., & Calabrese, J. R. (2001). Rapid, continuous cycling and psychiatric co-morbidity in pediatric bipolar I disorder. *Bipolar Disorders, 3*(4), 202–210.

Fristad, M. A., & Goldberg-Arnold, J. S. (2003). Family interventions for early-onset bipolar disorder. In B. G. Geller & M. P. DelBello (Eds.), *Bipolar Disorder in Childhood and Early Adolescence* (pp. 295–313). New York: Guilford Press.

Fristad, M. A., Verducci, J. S., Walters, K., & Young, M. E. (2009). Impact of multifamily psychoeducational psychotherapy in treating children aged 8 to 12 years with mood disorders. *Archives of General Psychiatry, 66*(9), 1013–1021.

Garrett, A. S., Reiss, A. L., Howe, M. E., Kelley, R. G., Singh, M. K., Adleman, N. E., . . . Chang, K. D. (2012). Abnormal amygdala and prefrontal cortex activation to facial expressions in pediatric bipolar disorder. *Journal of the American Academy of Child and Adolescent Psychiatry, 51*(8), 821–831.

Geller, B., Bolhofner, K., Craney, J. L., Williams, M., DelBello, M. P., & Gundersen, K. (2000). Psychosocial functioning in a prepubertal and early adolescent bipolar disorder phenotype. *Journal of the American Academy of Child and Adolescent Psychiatry, 39*(12), 1543–1548.

Geller, B., Craney, J. L., Bolhofner, K., Nickelsburg, M. J., Williams, M., & Zimerman, B. (2002). Two-year prospective follow-up of children with a prepubertal and early adolescent bipolar disorder phenotype. *American Journal of Psychiatry, 159*(6), 927–933.

Geller, B., Williams, M., Zimerman, B., Frazier, J., Beringer, L., & Warner, K. L. (1998). Prepubertal and early adolescent bipolarity differentiate from ADHD by manic symptoms, grandiose delusions, ultra-rapid or ultradian cycling. *Journal of Affective Disorders, 51*(2), 81–91.

Goldstein, T. R., Fersch-Podrat, R. K., Rivera, M., Axelson, D. A., Merranko, J., Yu, H., . . . Birmaher, B. (2015). Dialectical behavior therapy for adolescents with bipolar disorder: Results from a pilot randomized trial. *Journal of Child and Adolescent Psychopharmacology, 25*(2), 140–149.

Goldstein, T. R., Miklowitz, D. J., & Mullen, K. L. (2006). Social skills knowledge and performance among adolescents with bipolar disorder. *Bipolar Disorders, 8*(4), 350–361.

Greene, R. W. (2001). *The Explosive Child.* New York: Harper Collins Publishing.

Henin, A., Mick, E., Biederman, J., Fried, R., Wozniak, J., Faraone, S. V., . . . Doyle, A. E. (2007). Can bipolar disorder-specific neuropsychological impairments in children be identified? *Journal of Consulting and Clinical Psychology, 75*(2), 210.

Hlastala, S. A., Kotler, J. S., McClellan, J. M., & McCauley, E. A. (2010). Interpersonal and social rhythm therapy for adolescents with bipolar disorder: Treatment development and results from an open trial. *Depression and Anxiety, 27*(5), 457–464.

Keenan-Miller, D., Peris, T., Axelson, D., Kowatch, R. A., & Miklowitz, D. J. (2012). Family functioning, social impairment, and symptoms among adolescents with bipolar disorder. *Journal of the American Academy of Child and Adolescent Psychiatry, 51*(10), 1085–1094.

Kim, E. Y., Miklowitz, D. J., Biuckians, A., & Mullen, K. (2007). Life stress and the course of early-onset bipolar disorder. *Journal of Affective Disorders, 99*(1), 37–44.

Mayberg, H. S. (1997). *Limbic-cortical dysregulation. The Neuropsychiatry of Limbic and Subcortical Disorders* (pp. 167–178). American Psychiatric Press: Washington, DC.

Miklowitz, D. J., Axelson, D. A., Birmaher, B., George, E. L., Taylor, D. O., Schneck, C. D., . . . Brent, D. A. (2008). Family-focused treatment for adolescents with bipolar disorder: Results of a 2-year randomized trial. *Archives of General Psychiatry, 65*(9), 1053–1061.

Miklowitz, D. J., George, E. L., Axelson, D. A., Kim, E. Y., Birmaher, B., Schneck, C., . . . Brent, D. A. (2004). Family-focused treatment for adolescents with bipolar disorder. *Journal of Affective Disorders, 82,* S113–S128.

Passarotti, A. M., & Pavuluri, M. N. (2011). Brain functional domains inform therapeutic interventions in attention-deficit/hyperactivity disorder and pediatric bipolar disorder. *Expert Review of Neurotherapeutics, 11*(6), 897–914.

Pavuluri, M. N., Birmaher, B., & Naylor, M. (2005). Pediatric Bipolar Disorder: Ten year review. *Journal of the American Academy of Child and Adolescent Psychiatry, 44*(9), 846–871. PMID16113615.

Pavuluri, M. N., Graczyk, P. A., Henry, D. B., Carbray, J. A., Heidenreich, J., & Miklowitz, D. J. (2004). Child-and family-focused cognitive-behavioral therapy for pediatric bipolar disorder: Development and preliminary results. *Journal of the American Academy of Child and Adolescent Psychiatry, 43*(5), 528–537.

Pavuluri, M. N., Schenkel, L. S., Aryal, S., Harral, E. M., Hill, S. K., Herbener, E. S., & Sweeney, J. A. (2006). Neurocognitive function in unmedicated manic and medicated euthymic pediatric bipolar patients. *American Journal of Psychiatry, 163*(2), 286–293.

Rich, B. A., Carver, F. W., Holroyd, T., Rosen, H. R., Mendoza, J. K., Cornwell, B. R., . . . Leibenluft, E. (2011). Different neural pathways to negative affect in youth with pediatric bipolar disorder and severe mood dysregulation. *Journal of Psychiatric Research, 45*(10), 1283–1294.

Rucklidge, J. J. (2006). Psychosocial functioning of adolescents with and without paediatric bipolar disorder. *Journal of Affective Disorders, 91*(2), 181–188.

Schenkel, L. S., West, A. E., Harral, E. M., Patel, N. B., & Pavuluri, M. N. (2008). Parent–child interactions in pediatric bipolar disorder. *Journal of Clinical Psychology, 64*(4), 422–437.

Segal, Z., Williams, J., & Teasdale, J. (2002). *Mindfulness-Based Cognitive Therapy for Depression: A New Approach to Relapse Prevention.* New York: Guilford.

Weinstein, S. M., Henry, D., Katz, A, Peters, A. T., & West, A. E. (2015). Treatment moderators of child-and family-focused cognitive-behavioral therapy for pediatric bipolar disorder. *Journal of the American Academy of Child & Adolescent Psychiatry, 54.2,* 116–125.

West, A. E., Henry, D. B., & Pavuluri, M. N. (2007). Maintenance model of integrated psychosocial treatment in pediatric bipolar disorder: A pilot feasibility study. *Journal of the American Academy of Child and Adolescent Psychiatry, 46*(2), 205–212.

West, A. E., Jacobs, R. H., Westerholm, R., Lee, A., Carbray, J., Heidenreich, J., & Pavuluri, M. N. (2009). Child and family-focused cognitive-behavioral therapy for pediatric bipolar disorder: Pilot study of group treatment format. *Journal of the Canadian Academy of Child and Adolescent Psychiatry, 18*(3), 239–246.

West, A. E., & Pavuluri, M. N. (2009). Psychosocial treatments for childhood and adolescent bipolar disorder. *Child and Adolescent Psychiatric Clinics of North America, 18*(2), 471–482.

West, A. E., & Weinstein, S. M. (2011). A family-based psychosocial treatment model. *The Israel Journal of Psychiatry and Related Sciences, 49*(2), 86–93.

West, A. E., Weinstein, S. M., Peters, A. T., Katz, A. C., Henry, D. B., Cruz, R. A., & Pavuluri, M. N. (2014). Child- and family-focused cognitive-behavioral therapy for pediatric bipolar disorder: A randomized clinical trial. *Journal of the American Academy of Child and Adolescent Psychiatry, 53*(11), 1168–1178. e1161.

Wilens, T. E., Biederman, J., Forkner, P., Ditterline, J., Morris, M., Moore, H., . . . Wozniak, J. (2003). Patterns of comorbidity and dysfunction in clinically referred preschool and school-age children with bipolar disorder. *Journal of Child and Adolescent Psychopharmacology, 13*(4), 495–505.

Wozniak, J., Biederman, J., Kiely, K., Ablon, J. S., Faraone, S. V., Mundy, E., & Mennin, D. (1995). Mania-like symptoms suggestive of childhood-onset bipolar disorder in clinically referred children. *Journal of the American Academy of Child and Adolescent Psychiatry, 34*(7), 867–876.

Yurgelun-Todd, D. A., Gruber, S. A., Kanayama, G., Killgore, W. D., Baird, A. A., & Young, A. D. (2000). fMRI during affect discrimination in bipolar affective disorder. *Bipolar Disorders, 2*, 237–248.

Introduction and Overview of RAINBOW Program

1. Introductions and goals for treatment
2. Introduce concept of RAINBOW treatment
3. Engagement issues
4. Pre-treatment measures
5. Relationship-building with the child
6. Summary and homework

Participants: Parents (or caregivers); child

Required materials: **Handouts #1–6**, pen

Session length: 75 minutes

Objective

This session's objective is to orient parents and the child to the RAINBOW treatment program and engage them in the treatment process.

Conceptual Background

The RAINBOW program was developed through a review of the literature and clinical experience relevant to the developmental psychopathology and treatment of pediatric bipolar disorder (PBD). The RAINBOW program is an accumulation of best practices for the psychosocial treatment of pediatric bipolar disorder. It is important at the beginning of this treatment program that you provide an overview of the program and establish a therapeutic alliance and shared goals between the families and you.

Activities Related to Objective

1. Introductions and Goals for Treatment (10 min.)

Introduce yourself and discuss treatment-related issues:

- Confidentiality
- Starting on time and ending on time
- Importance of everyone feeling comfortable enough to share
- Supporting each other throughout the process

Discuss the importance of setting goals:

- Ask the parents what they hope to get out of treatment
- Ask the child what he hopes to get out of treatment
- Help the family identify their key targets for intervention and behavior change (e.g., rage episodes, school performance, peer relationships)

2. Introduce the Concept of RAINBOW Treatment (20 min.)

> ✓ *Therapist Note: Key terms are underlined. Depending on the level of functioning of the family, you may want to spend extra time defining these terms for the parents and child.*

RAINBOW is a psychosocial treatment for parents and children developed to address factors associated with bipolar disorder in children that might make the illness worse (e.g., lack of self-esteem, overstressed parents, coping skills that don't work, or poor peer relationships). The foundation of RAINBOW is the *vulnerability-stress* model, which means that psychosocial *stressors* interact with the child's individual *genetic* and *biological predisposition* to make symptoms worse. We cannot change genetics, but we can help change the psychosocial functioning of the child and family to make symptoms better and help everybody function better—in relationships, at home, and in school.

Some aspects of the environment can serve as stressors, including stressful life events, poor peer relationships, lack of coping skills, and negative communication styles within families. *Psychoeducation, cognitive behavioral therapy*, and *interpersonal problem solving* are the specific techniques used in RAINBOW to help parents and children better understand and manage bipolar disorder.

RAINBOW has its theoretical foundation in three core areas of scientific findings:

- The unique characteristics of pediatric bipolar disorder (rapid cycling, chronicity, irritability, mixed depression, and comorbidity);
- Affective circuitry dysfunction (excessive reactivity of amygdala, underactivity in frontal cortex related to poor problem solving); and
- Environmental stressors (peer rejection, family conflict, low self-esteem/feelings of worthlessness, exhaustion and strain in parents, school problems)

This knowledge was considered in developing the seven main ingredients of RAINBOW.

✓ **Instructions:** *Distribute* **Handout #1** *to parent and child. Explain the concepts so that the family can easily understand.*

R: Routines

Evidence: Disturbances in routine can trigger or intensify mood dysregulation. Incorporation of pleasurable activities into a child's routine is important in treating mood problems.

Goal: Increase affect regulation and decrease symptoms' exacerbation by establishing a predictable, simplified routine.

A: Affect Regulation

Evidence: Neurobiological underpinnings of pediatric bipolar disorder make it difficult for these children to regulate their emotions.

Goal: Use of appropriate behavioral management and coping strategies to help regulate emotions.

I: I Can Do It!

Evidence: Sense of self-efficacy plays an important role in predicting the onset and recurrence of mood episodes.

Goal: Increase children's and parents' belief in their ability to cope with the disorder, and increase positive self-concept in children.

N: No Negative Thoughts, and Live in the Now

Evidence: Children with mood disorders have maladaptive cognitions and distortions in self-evaluation.

Goal: Decrease negative thinking and thought distortions in self-evaluation. Emphasize living in the present moment to avoid catastrophic thinking.

B: Be a Good Friend, and Balanced Lifestyle for Parents

Evidence: Children with bipolar disorder often have significant difficulties in peer relationships.

Goal: Improve social functioning in children. For parents, develop a more balanced lifestyle that involves finding ways to replenish their energy and enjoy life.

O: Oh, How Can We Solve the Problem?

Evidence: Problem-solving skills are impaired in children with bipolar disorder.

Goal: Teach effective and collaborative problem-solving to children and parents.

W: Ways to Get Support

Evidence: Isolation, shame, and lack of access can prevent children with bipolar disorder and parents from finding support systems.

Goal: Help identify and seek out support systems for the child and parents—family, school, community.

3. Engagement Issues (15 min.)

Explain the importance of engagement in treatment and address the following topics, which may increase your clients' understanding of the therapeutic process and optimize session attendance.

"Culture" of This Treatment

- Active involvement by the parent, child, and you is required.
- Change occurs through practice, which the parent(s) and child do outside of the session.
- You provide clinical knowledge based on your training and your work with families. Parents are the experts on their child and how well techniques will work in their lives.

- This is a collaborative process, and there is no "magic bullet." The idea is to work together. Some things may work, others may not.
- The parents should feel comfortable letting you know when things are working well and when things aren't working. Together, you and the parents can figure out how to make the strategies work.

Structure of Treatment

- Sessions take place for 12 weeks. Sessions are of variable lengths. Most child and family sessions are 60 minutes long. Parent-only sessions are 90 minutes.
- Each session has a main goal for the child and/or the parent to help learn strategies to manage the disorder and to feel more "in charge."
- The child and parents are taught strategies and given the opportunity to practice in-session and between sessions. The parents and you should take a collaborative approach so that parents can pick strategies that they feel comfortable using.

Parental Attitudes/Attributions

Assess if the parent understands, agrees with, and/or has questions about RAINBOW. There are several thoughts or feelings parents may have regarding their involvement in RAINBOW. Since RAINBOW is an adjunctive treatment to pharmacological intervention, parents may assume that medication is the only type of intervention necessary to treat children with bipolar disorder. Because of PBD's "biological" and "genetic" underpinnings, parents may not understand the importance of psychosocial interventions beyond medication intervention. The goal for today is to assess for this, not to change or challenge these beliefs.

Parental Expectations

Help parents understand what they can reasonably expect from treatment:

- Change takes time. The child (and parents) have had years of interacting with each other in a certain way. Treatment focuses on helping the child and parents interact differently with each other and with other people. It will take time for parents to learn new skills, and it will take time for the child to respond differently.
- Behavior typically gets worse before it gets better. Nobody likes change. As parents try new things, the child will "test" them to see if the parents "mean it."

- There are a lot of influences on the child which the parents may not be able to control. Some kids have difficult temperaments or have language or learning difficulties that make it harder for a parent to raise the child. Parents cannot control these things, but they can, through the way they interact with their child, lessen their impact on the child's behavior.
- There will be times when parents and their child will be making progress and then will have a setback. This is not a linear process.

Child's Expectations

Ask the child to explain his ideas about why he is here today. What does he think treatment is going to be like? Does he have worries? Is there anything he is looking forward to about this process?

Obstacles to Treatment

Help parents anticipate obstacles to participation, and problem-solve about what can be done to minimize the impact of these obstacles. It may be necessary to have an open discussion about the length of treatment by discussing each of the following issues and how they may affect the family's attendance and fidelity to treatment.

External obstacles include:

- Transportation
- Other family members that might make it difficult for parents to attend
- Housing issues
- Babysitting or childcare
- Other commitments

Internal obstacles include:

- Parent doesn't believe it will help
- Too much work when parent has a lot of demands
- This isn't the way parent wants to parent

4. Completing Pre-treatment Measures (Optional, Pending Therapist Preference)

Explain the importance of tracking progress and understanding how participation in RAINBOW impacts symptoms and functioning. Then hand out measures and give parents instructions.

5. Relationship-Building with the Child (20 min.)

Why Am I Here? Game

To play this game, use your judgement based on the child's age. For younger children (typically those who 10 or younger), attach **Handout #2** (three pieces of paper labeled YES, NO, and NOT SURE) to the wall, apart from each other. Then ask the child questions from the "Why Am I Here?" question sheet (**Handout #3**). For children 11 and older, it may be more appropriate to verbally discuss the questions. In either case, explain that there are no right or wrong answers, and what matters most is what the child thinks. However, when discussing the "bad" and "in trouble" questions, remind the child that she is not in therapy because of being bad or in trouble. For each question, have the child go to the paper that fits his response. Ask follow-up questions after the child has made her choice. Compliment the child for sharing.

Interview Activity

In this activity, the child and you take turns interviewing each other using the "Getting to Know You" interview sheet (**Handout #4**). When done, the child and you report to each other what you each have learned about the other person. Explain that you are going to collect the interview and put it in the "Rainbow Treasures" folder that will contain all of the activities the child completes during the course of the treatment.

6. Summary and Homework (10 min.)

Summary

Briefly review and summarize today's session: RAINBOW was developed through a review of the literature and clinical experience. The acronym

"RAINBOW" represents the seven main ingredients of the program. As with any program, it is the sum of the parts of the program rather than any one concept within the program that will affect the long-term course of the disorder. That is why their engagement and their attendance at every session are important. Ask if the parents have questions regarding anything that was discussed today.

Homework for the Parents

Ask the parents to think during the week of any questions they have regarding pediatric bipolar disorder or its treatment; write them down, and bring the questions to the next session, which will focus on psychoeducation.

Homework for the Child

Give the child the "Feelings Poster" (**Handout #5**) and "My Feeling Today Is" (**Handout #6**). Explain that he is to pick a time over the upcoming week to complete the "My Feeling Today Is" sheet, and encourage him to use the "Feelings Poster" to help identify how he is feeling. Explain that if he brings back the completed "My Feeling Today Is" sheet next week, he will receive a small prize at the end of session (e.g., small snack/candy, colorful pencil). Explain that, unlike in school, "late work" can be brought back for full credit, and that even if he forgets to bring back his Feeling Exercise at the next session, he can complete it and bring it back another time and receive a prize then (in addition to any other Feeling Exercise that he has completed on time).

However, discourage the child from saving all his Feeling Exercises to turn in until the last session in order to receive many prizes, as the purpose of the Feeling Exercises is to help learn to identify feelings, as well as their causes and effects, and to facilitate the sharing of feelings.

RAINBOW Notebook

Explain to the parents and child that all homework, worksheets, and activities completed during the 12-week session will be compiled into a RAINBOW Binder for the child to keep after treatment.

Psychoeducation about Pediatric Bipolar Disorder

A: Affect Regulation

AGENDA

1. Review materials covered in last session
2. "How was your week?" Review homework
3. Psychoeducation on pediatric bipolar disorder
4. RAINBOW skill: introduction to mood charting
5. Summary and homework

Participants: Parents (or caregivers); child

Required materials: **Handouts #7–10**, prize basket, pen

Session length: 75 minutes

1. Review Materials from Last Session, Briefly (5 min.)

The previous session introduced the components of the RAINBOW treatment program and discussed engagement issues. Briefly review these topics and see if the parents and/or the child have any questions.

2. Review Homework and Discuss How the Past Week Went (5 min.)

Review homework from last week and tell the child that she will get a prize at end of session, if the homework has been completed.

3. Psychoeducation on Pediatric Bipolar Disorder (30 min.)

> ✓ *Instructions: Hand out the psychoeducation information packet to parents and child (**Handout #7**). Some of the language may be overly advanced or technical for the child to understand. Explain big concepts to the child throughout the psychoeducation process in easier-to-understand language. Engage the child in the presentation by assigning the role to the child to place a star on the printed pages of the slides that the child finds to be helpful.*

Objective

This session's objective is to provide parents information on the incidence, prevalence, assessment, presentation, diagnosis, and course of pediatric bipolar disorder.

Conceptual Background

There is considerable information about pediatric bipolar disorder from a variety of sources that have varying empirical support. The packet of slides and subsequent discussion are meant to clarify information for parents and allow them an opportunity to better understand the current state of the research in this area. However, this information is meant to be personalized by each parent. It is important for parents to understand how this information applies to their child and how to use this information to better understand the presentation and course of their child's illness.

Activities Related to Objective

Psychoeducation Packet

Go through the psychoeducation packet (**Handout #7**), page by page, explaining the concepts to the parents and child. Allow the parents and child to ask questions as you go along.

Open the psychoeducational session by asking general questions to elicit parents' thoughts about their personal experiences with pediatric bipolar disorder. For example:

- What is pediatric bipolar disorder?
- What does pediatric bipolar disorder look like?
- What are the common symptoms of pediatric bipolar disorder?
- When discussing symptoms, pay close attention to what your child presents. What are the top symptoms to target in treatment for your child?

Slide 1: Introduction to pediatric bipolar disorder

Slide 2: Discuss the concept of the vulnerability-stress model of illness

Individuals present with unique genetic, biological, and psychological predispositions. In addition, there are socioenvironmental stressors (e.g., peer relationships, academic stress). These factors often interact. The extent to which these interactions produce positive or negative outcomes is affected by both protective and risk factors. One goal of RAINBOW is for the family to understand what these factors are for each child and family, and how best to manage these factors in order to maximize positive outcomes.

- Predispositions: genetic transmission (50% of pediatric bipolar disorder is accounted for genetically)
- Protective factors: caring family, good communication style, healthy parents, early identification
- Risk factors: several biological teratogens (alcohol exposure); low IQ; low competence

Slide 3: Mood spectrum chart

Present this slide to describe the full range of emotion in individuals.

- Many fall into the "normal range"—middle
- Moods on the spectrum:
  - Depression—more chronically sad (blue)
  - Dysthymia—mostly blue but not Major Depressive Disorder (MDD)
  - Hypomania—driven, not a lot of rest
  - Mania—over-the-top elation, hypersexuality, grandiosity, overactivity

- Disorders on the spectrum:
  - Cyclothymia—running the range from dysthymia–hypomania
  - Bipolar II—more depressive (more MDD than anything)
  - Bipolar I—severe manic/MDD
  - Unspecified Bipolar Disorder—classification for individuals who do not fit nicely into other categories
- Diagnosis depends on where their symptoms fall on this spectrum, and functional impairment over a long period of time

Slide 4: Brief overview of pediatric bipolar disorder

Pediatric Bipolar Disorder is a mood disorder with episodes of mania, depression, or mixed elements of both, and associated symptoms.

- Bipolar Spectrum: Type I, II, Unspecified subtypes
- Severity, duration of episodes-contribute to-diagnosis

Pediatric bipolar disorder is a "brain" disorder that causes excessive emotional reactivity and difficulty with problem-solving and using cognitive functions during excessive emotional states. It has unique features compared to adult-onset.

Slides 5–6: What is pediatric bipolar disorder?

Core features are either elevated/expansive mood OR irritable mood (or both). Explain the difference. Provide descriptors for mood states in children and examples from children and families living with pediatric bipolar disorder. Discuss mood states with parents and ask which of these are seen in their child.

Slides 7–13: Pediatric bipolar disorder symptoms and examples from clinical work with children

Discuss each slide with the parents, initiating discussion about their own experience with these different symptoms and whether the examples resonate with their experience.

Slide 14: Typical and associated symptoms of depression

Slide 15: Neurobiological underpinnings that make pharmacotherapy useful—activation of amygdala with negative emotion

Slide 16: Unique characteristics of pediatric bipolar disorder

Slide 17: Concept of cycling in pediatric bipolar disorder—including a description of daily or "ultradian" cycling

What is this notion of cycling? It involves moving from one mood state to another.

- Mood calendar will help the parents to understand cycling (will be discussed later)
- Cycling (going from happy/elated to depressed/irritable/withdrawn)
- Cycles can be called *mood swings, episodes*

  - Children tend to cycle more than adults
  - Adults have clearer, more distinct cycles
  - Children have more cycling, and it is less distinct
  - There are many different terms used to describe children who cycle (*ultracycling, ultradian, rapid cycling, mood swings, episodes*)
  - It is important for parents to think of shifts and patterns that could help explain temporal onset of illness
  - It is important to keep reminders or a journal to help with treatment. This also helps with identifying specific problems to focus on in treatment

Slide 18: Comorbidity

Three common diagnoses that are often comorbid with pediatric bipolar disorder are Attention-Deficit/Hyperactivity Disorder (ADHD), Oppositional Defiant Disorder (ODD), and Anxiety Disorders.

Slide 19: Psychotic symptoms may also be present in children with pediatric bipolar disorder

Go through each symptom and ask parents about their child's experience with each.

Slide 20: Illustration of integrated evidence-based practice

Slide 21: Website for the under Depression and Bipolar Support Alliance (DBSA)—a good resource

Slide 22: Website for National Alliance on Mental Illness (NAMI)—a good resource

Slide 23: There is hope—this is a treatable illness!

Signature Symptoms (5 min.)

It can be helpful for the parents and child to identify what they consider the "signature" symptoms of the disorder in this particular child. For example, for some children it's rage episodes, for others it's over-the-top silliness, -and- for others it's weepiness. Identifying the "signature" for this child can help the parents and the child give a name to their most troubling symptoms. Some parents and children even come up with a name for their child's signature symptoms (some we've heard in the past include: "meltdown," "volcano," "Bob"). The identification of the primary concerning symptoms can also help drive priorities in treatment.

Importance of Medication (10 min.)

Use the Medication Discussion Questions sheet (**Handout #8**) in order to explore the parents' and child's perceptions of positive and negative aspects of medication, tips for compliance, ways doctors and parents can help, and other relevant medication-related topics. Encourage the child to participate, to provide her honest feelings, and let her know that her opinion is valued. In addition to soliciting her thoughts and feelings about medication, a second goal is to help the child and parents realize that others are going through similar situations and to normalize taking medication for bipolar disorder. You should stress the importance of consistent medication compliance, the fact that each individual may have a different response to the same medication, and that it may take numerous attempts for the doctor to find the right medication(s) for the child.

4. RAINBOW Skill: Establish Mood Charts for Children

Objective

The goal is to assist the parent and the child in being able to reliably monitor and track the child's mood and the associated environmental antecedents and consequences.

Conceptual Background

Behaviors and emotions often have antecedents and consequences associated with their occurrence. For example, certain times of the day, particular activities, or particular people may be antecedents to the occurrence of irritable moods in children. Likewise, consequences such as getting out of doing an unpreferred activity or obtaining attention from adults may also be associated with certain behavior or moods. Children may exhibit fluctuations in their mood depending on other observable factors, such as certain days (the early part of the school week) or months of the year (winter months). In order to understand the relationship between moods and behavior, and to plan for and implement treatment over the long term, tracking such patterns in the expression of mood and behavior is important. Monitoring is ideally done by both the parent and the child.

Activities Related to Objective

Discussion about Mood Monitoring (5 min.)

Discuss the concept of antecedents and consequences of behaviors and moods, and the importance of recognizing patterns.

We are often not aware of how we are feeling and how those feelings affect the way we behave or react. Learning to identify our moods can help make us more aware of how we're feeling in the moment and be aware of when we may be likely to react or behave in maladaptive ways due to difficult feelings.

Monitoring also helps us see if there are patterns in the child's feelings or moods or certain situations that cause her to feel a certain ways. By doing this, we can try to learn ways to decrease difficult feelings and increase pleasant feelings (e.g., sleep maintenance, predictable routine, limiting interpersonal stressors). However, it is important to stress the fact that there is nothing wrong with experiencing "difficult" feelings (e.g., anger, irritability, sadness), and that the goal is to learn how to express those feelings adaptively and prosocially.

As an example, ask the parent and child to discuss the signature symptom(s) they identified previously in this session and to brainstorm or identify possible antecedents and consequences for the symptom(s).

Introduce the parent and child to the Mood Calendar (**Handout #9**). Explain to them that they will be asked to complete mood calendars each week for every week of treatment. (Be sure to provide enough copies of the handout.) Instruct the parents and child to rate the child's mood three times each day, using the color-coded system on the calendar. Explain that they can also add colors and moods if there are ones not represented on the form.

Discuss the importance of mood monitoring with child. Encourage him to complete each section of the chart (i.e., morning, afternoon, and evening) as close to that time period as possible, as opposed to waiting until the end of the day or the end of the week, so that he will have less difficulty accurately remembering how he felt. This may be accomplished by bringing the chart to school each day in his binder or homework folder, or placing it in a prominent position at home (e.g., on the refrigerator).

Engage the child and parent in completing the mood calendar for today to guide the child through the process and to identify any barriers to understanding.

5. Summary and Homework (5 min.)

Summary

It is important to understand what we know about pediatric bipolar disorder and what the science tells us. There is a lot of misinformation out there. Encourage the parents and child to continue to ask questions as they come up. Mood monitoring is an essential aspect of treatment as it helps the child, parents, and therapist recognize patterns in mood dysregulation, as well as to identify antecedents, or triggers, for mood fluctuations.

Homework for the Parents

Parents have two assignments for next session. First, they are asked to identify three symptoms that their child exhibits. Have the parents discuss the symptoms with their child. Does the child call the symptom by the same name as the parent? It is important for the parent and child to develop a language that is common that can be used within the family and in treatment. Questions for the parent include: How do you talk to your child about this? What does your child call it? What is a common language to describe it? Second, ask the parents to complete their own mood calendar for the child for the week (**Handout #9**), as well as help the child to complete his for the next two weeks, as the child will not be at the next session.

Homework for the Child

The child should complete the mood calendar for the next two weeks (next week's session is parents only). The child should rate her mood three times every day according to instructions on the mood calendar. If the child brings her completed sheets to the next session (in two weeks), she will receive a small prize at the end of that session.

✓ *Instructions:* *Let the child pick a prize at the end of this session for completion of last session's homework. Give out the "Try at Home!" sheet (**Handout #10**) for this session.*

Affect Regulation Skills for Parents

RAINBOW INGREDIENTS

R: Routine
A: Affect Regulation

AGENDA

1. Review materials covered in last session
2. "How was your week?" Review homework
3. RAINBOW skills: affect regulation for parents
   a. Establishing routines for children
   b. Acknowledging difficult feelings and acceptance
   c. Affect regulation: helping children identify feelings
   d. Anger management and modeling appropriate responses
4. Summary and homework

Participants: Parents (or caregivers)

Required materials: **Handouts #11–12**, pen

Session length: 90 minutes

1. Review Materials Covered in the Last Session (5 min.)

Did any questions come up about psychoeducational materials from last session?

2. Discuss How the Week Went and Process any Issues or Problems that Came Up; Review Homework (5 min.)

Ask the parents how the discussion on identifying and labeling symptoms went with their child. Did the parents or child have any difficulties establishing common language around symptoms?

Review the parents' mood calendar and discuss any problems, questions, and things that were helpful about completing it.

3. RAINBOW Skills

a. Establish Routines for Children (15 min.)

Objective

To help parents establish predictable, simplified routines that will reduce excessive reactivity and tense negotiations in response to changes in the child's schedule.

Conceptual Background

Children engage in a variety of activities throughout the day. Ideally, routines are established for these activities so children have clear expectations regarding these activities. Having clear expectations allows children to modulate their behavior and emotions regarding these daily activities and reduces frustration arising from unexpected occurrences. In addition, some routines are important for overall emotional and behavioral functioning (e.g., sleep and nutrition), such that disruption in these routines can have dramatic effects on children's functioning throughout the day. For children who have difficulties with affect, emotion, and behavior, routines are of utmost importance. In this session, a goal is to identify areas where routines are important to establish, discuss potential routines within these areas, and to monitor routines to determine the effectiveness of routines for daily functioning.

Activities Related to Objective

1. Ask the parents about important daily activities in which their child participates or is involved in (e.g., getting ready for the day in the morning, going to and attending school, exercise, play time, homework, chores, nutrition, sleep, medicine).

2. Discuss the importance of managing their child's emotions related to making transitions (e.g., transitioning from playing to going to bed at night; transitioning from the breakfast table to the school bus in the morning). Transitions can be very difficult for children with bipolar disorder and can trigger mood dysregulation. To the extent possible, transitions should be predictable, made into a daily routine, and come with plenty of warning and preparation.

3. Using **Handout #11,** help parents identify important activities to target for routines with their own child, and brainstorm ways to establish these routines (e.g., nutrition, making sure the child drinks enough water, sleep, making sure child goes to bed at an appropriate time). Identify ways to implement routines family-wide (i.e., for all children in the household).

4. Discuss with the parents how best to communicate these routines to their children and getting children's input on these routines.

5. Discuss with the parents why it is important to have routines and how to monitor these routines (e.g., posted schedules, reminders).

b. Acknowledge Difficult Feelings in Parents (15 min.)

Objective

The objective is to normalize parent's range of emotions regarding their child and provide them with an opportunity to recognize and accept these feelings in a supportive environment.

Conceptual Background

Parenting is a daunting task; parenting a child with a mood disorder can seem overwhelming. Parents may experience a range of different emotions about their child and their child's mood disorder. It is important to acknowledge and process these feelings in order to work through their impact on their family system. Parents may feel *shame* or *embarrassment* about their child's behavior or may feel *confused* about how to manage their child's moods. They may feel *angry* or *exasperated* with their child, or *fearful* about what the future holds for their child. Parents also may feel *scared* and *desperate* for help. Or they may feel *pained* by their child's feelings of depression and hopelessness. Finally, parents may experience *guilt* about their potential role in their child's distress and harbor deep-seated *worries* that they are somehow at fault for their child's suffering.

It is important for parents to embrace the concept of *acceptance* in thinking about their child's disorder. Acceptance that their child did not "choose" to have a mood disorder and does not "choose" to feel or behave the way he does-can alleviate some of the frustration and the power struggles that are likely to occur. If parents assume that the child's moods and ensuing behavior may be out of his control, then they can work with the child to support and guide him, rather than becoming angry or trying to punish their child into behaving appropriately.

Activities Related to Objective

1. Provide the parents with an opportunity to discuss the feelings they have about their child and their child's mood disorder.
2. Encourage parents to talk about particular experiences or situations that trigger some of these feelings.
3. Validate that all these emotions are normal reactions to the parents' experience and that having negative feelings about their own child does not make them bad parents.
4. Discuss the concept of acceptance with parents. Children with bipolar disorder cannot always control their behavior, and it is difficult for parents to grasp this concept sometimes—they want to believe that their child could behave differently if she chose to. Discuss how parent roles can change from "punisher" to "coach" when the parents assume that the child cannot control her behavior. Explain that this is an ongoing process and not something parents can achieve immediately.

c. Affect regulation—Helping Children Identify Difficult Feelings (20 min.)

Objective

The objective is to help parents think of ways that they can help their child develop a language for the child's different mood states and feelings, and to help their child identify and communicate these feelings to the parents.

Conceptual Background

Children have a range of different mood states and feelings that accompany this disorder, including, but not limited to, anger, frustration, hurt, sadness, disappointment, and fear. Depending on the child's age, developmental level, and previous experiences, he may not have the language or skills necessary to identify and name these feelings when they come up. Being able to identify feelings is an important first step in coping with them and asking others for help. Therefore, developing a language for emotions and skills in identifying and communicating them to others is an important aspect of treatment.

Activities Related to Objective

1. Discuss with the parents the importance of helping their child develop a language for his different feelings and being able to identify and communicate them to his parents and others.
2. Help parents brainstorm and name some of the different emotions they think their child routinely feels.
3. Help parents think of ways to increase these skills in their child, such as encouraging the child to name his feelings; reflecting back to the child how they think he must be feeling; encouraging the child to use "feeling words" to express himself; and using books or games to increase the child's emotional vocabulary.

d. Anger Management and Modeling Appropriate Responses (20 min.)

Objective

The objective is to help parents develop more effective ways to cope with their child's angry feelings and behavioral outbursts. Another goal is to help parents to have a neutral expression and speak in a low-pitched tone of voice while expressing calming yet appropriate words during a time when the child is exhibiting excessive emotions.

Conceptual Background

Children with bipolar disorder often experience intense anger and explosive rage episodes that are overwhelming and frustrating for parents. One important thing for parents to remember is that, during these episodes, their child may feel like she has no control over her feelings. Therefore, intervening with limits or consequences immediately may be ineffective and potentially exacerbate the episode. The most immediate priority should be to help the child calm down and use her coping skills. It is a good idea for parents and their child to work together to come up with a detailed coping plan for these episodes with specific steps for parents and the child to follow. Some children may need to be soothed, while others may need "space." Therefore, the plan will need to be individualized to each child. Consequences for behavior that occurred during the episode may still be necessary, but they should be implemented after the episode has occurred and the child is calm. Consequences should be firm, with no negotiation, and parents should ALWAYS follow through after they have established a consequence. Otherwise, their child will learn the message that consequences do not mean anything, and she will continue to test these limits.

In addition, excessive expression of emotion by children can be very stressful for parents to manage. Parents may inadvertently intensify the situation by their own emotional reaction to their child or the manner in which the parent attempts to solve the situation. In many cases, any attempt by the parents to remedy the situation by increasing their own expression of emotion, or by attempting to implement consequences, often worsens the situation. Typically, the best course for parents is to remain neutral and to assist the child in managing her own mood by speaking in a low-pitched tone of voice while expressing calming yet appropriate words. Addressing the expressed emotion is important, but this should typically be done after the emotional episode is over.

Activities Related to Objective

A "fire" analogy may be used to highlight the session's objective; namely, the importance of de-escalation and containment during a child's rage episode, versus the enforcement of consequences, punishment, or parental expression of emotion. To help make this concept concrete, engage the parent in a discussion of appropriate responses to a *fire in the household*.

1. What would the family do in the event of a fire? (e.g., contain the fire, establish the safety of all family members, and attempt to put out the fire). During a fire, one would NOT engage with the fire, watch the fire, try to figure out how the fire started or who is responsible, discuss how upsetting the fire is or what to do to prevent the next fire, etc.—that would not be safe or helpful!
   - Likewise, a child's rage episodes should be treated similarly—the priority is to help the child calm down and contain the child ("put out the fire") while establishing the safety of all family members. Then, *only once* the fire has been put out and the episode has defused can the family engage in a discussion of consequences and prevention.

- Parents should be encouraged to recall this analogy (e.g., through use of mantras—"Put out the fire," or visual images of a fire, smoke, or putting on fireman gear) during rage episodes to help both parent and child de-escalate and remain calm.

2. Give the parents an opportunity to speak about how scary and frustrating these rage episodes can be.

3. Ask the parents to describe the last time their child exhibited excessive emotion and discuss what it was like for them.

4. Ask the parents what they typically do in reaction to these kinds of situations. What has worked? What hasn't worked? (Typically, parents should be able to identify that trying to equal their child's expressed emotion or to immediately remedy the situation through punishment does not work.)

5. Explain that when a child with bipolar disorder gets this angry, he may feel totally out of control, and the first priority will be to help him calm down and regain control over the situation. This should be done in an empathic and planned-out way.

6. Explain that once the episode is diffused and everyone is calm, then consequences for negative behavior can be implemented. This will be more effective than trying to implement a consequence when the child is experiencing rage and completely out of control.

7. Assist parents in identifying ways to remain neutral and calm (identifying coping words and phrases, paced breathing, distraction) that can be implemented during these situations. This provides important modeling of appropriate anger responses.

8. Encourage parents to sit down with their child and develop a coping plan for these episodes, which will include a step-by-step plan for both the child and parents. Brainstorm with parents some ideas for these coping plans.

4. Summary and Homework (10 min.)

Summary

Summarize the importance of routines, identifying activities that require routines, establishing routines for these activities, and discussing routines with children.

- Review the importance of parents' learning to acknowledge and accept their own difficult feelings, and ask them to practice doing this over the upcoming weeks.
- Review strategies parents can use to help their child recognize and identify her feelings.
- Review strategies to help diffuse extreme anger episodes, and techniques parents can use to remain calm themselves.

Homework for the Parents

Parents should pick one, or several, areas that they think are important for their child in terms of establishing a routine (meals, bedtime, etc.) and commit to establishing a strict routine and discussing it with their child.

Parents should also commit to trying a few strategies over the course of the week to help their child identify feelings, such as reading him a feelings book, helping him name an emotion, or helping him fill out a "My feeling today is . . ." sheet.

Parents should also commit to trying to use different approaches to handling their child's anger and modeling appropriate responses if an anger episode occurs over the course of the next week.

✓ *Instructions:* Give out the "Try at Home!" sheet (**Handout #12**) for this session.

**Affect Regulation Skills
for Children**

A: Affect Regulation

1. Review materials covered in last session
2. "How was your week?" Review homework
3. RAINBOW skills: recognizing and understanding emotions
   a. Recognizing and labeling emotions
   b. Recognizing difficult feelings
   c. Recognizing triggers
4. Summary and homework

Participants: Child only; check in with the parents at the end of the session

Required materials: **Handouts #9** and **#13–18**, prize basket, pen

Session length: 60 minutes

1. Review Materials Covered in the Last Session (5 min.)

Ask if the child has any questions or remembers what was discussed in the last session.

2. Discuss How the Last Two Weeks Went and Process Any Issues or Problems that Came Up; Review Homework (10 min.)

Review the child's mood calendar and discuss any problems, questions, and things that were helpful about completing it. Remind the child that she will get a prize at the end of the session for each completed mood calendar that she has brought with her (two are possible, as it has been two weeks since your last session with this child). Questions to ask the child include:

- What was it like to try to keep track of your feelings each day?
- What was the most difficult part of completing the mood calendar?
- Did you find that you were feeling more than just one feeling at the same time?
- Were there certain events or situations that you think caused you to feel _____ (happy, sad, anxious, irritable, etc.)?
- Did you find any patterns in your feelings during the week?
- Did you find it too difficult to identify or remember what you were feeling when you were trying to complete the mood calendar?
- Why might it be important or useful to be able to complete the daily mood calendar?

Review the following points from the previous session: We are often not aware of how we are feeling and how those feelings affect the way we behave or react. Learning to identify our moods can help make us more aware of how we're feeling in the moment and to be aware of when we may be likely to react or behave in maladaptive ways due to difficult feelings.

Communicate to the child that using a mood calendar also helps us see if there are patterns in our feeling or moods or if certain situations cause us to feel certain ways. Developing this understanding will help us to learn ways to decrease difficult feelings and increase pleasant feelings. However, it is important to stress the fact that there is nothing wrong with experiencing "difficult" feelings (e.g., anger, irritability, sadness), and the goal is to learn how to express those feelings adaptively and prosocially.

Objective

The objective is to help the child to recognize and be able to label the range of different emotions he may feel, to normalize the experience of intense emotion, and to teach the child how to cope with intense negative emotion.

Conceptual Background

Children with bipolar disorder feel emotions very intensely. This can be scary and overwhelming for them, but there are methods for managing and coping with intense emotions that they can learn to make it less scary. The first step in being able to cope with extreme emotions is to be able to recognize and label feelings when they happen. Once children can identify their emotions, they can take measures to decrease their negative impact. Although they may not be able to prevent strong emotions from occurring, they can have a certain amount of control over what they do with the emotions when they arise. It is important for children to be able to recognize triggers for negative emotions so that they can either prevent these triggers or anticipate them. It is also important for them to have skills to cope with negative emotions that they cannot prevent, as the experience of a range of emotions is inevitable in daily life.

a. Recognizing and Labeling Emotions (8 min.)

> ✓ *Instructions: Provide the child with a RAINBOW picture (**Handout #13**) and have a discussion with her about how each element of the picture applies to the RAINBOW treatment and bipolar disorder symptoms. Engage the child by allowing her to color in the picture as you are discussing the various components, which will later become the cover for her RAINBOW binder.*

Activities Related to Objective

Emphasize each of the following picture-elements:

- *The rainbow:* The rainbow represents the spectrum of emotions that are experienced by everyone. Ask the child to think of emotions and how they may be represented in the rainbow. At a minimum, *sad, happy, angry, irritable, worried,* and *neutral/fair* should be mentioned. Discuss and normalize each of the different feelings or emotions. Although some emotions are more difficult to experience than others (e.g., anger, sadness, worry), everyone experiences the full spectrum of emotions, and it is that experience that makes us who we are. Then discuss the unique experience of moods or emotions in relation to pediatric bipolar disorder (e.g., rapid cycling, mixed mania, elation, depression).

- *The cloud/rain:* The cloud and the rain represent the difficult/ negative events and situations that occur in the life of the child.
- *The girl/umbrella:* Even though the girl is being rained on (i.e., enduring bad/negative events), she remains positive and is able to protect herself with her umbrella (i.e., the skills that she has acquired to deal with bipolar disorder and difficult situations, which will be learned and practiced in treatment). Thus, negative events can be overcome, despite the fact that they may seem overwhelming at the time.
- *The boy/dog:* The boy and his dog represent friendship, mutual caring, and responsibility. The positive aspects of these characteristics can be discussed as they apply to the child.
- *The sun:* The sun represents the positive events that occur in our life. Even though bad events (i.e., the cloud and rain) occur at times and may seem as though they will never end, positive events will also occur and help us maintain a sense of hopefulness.
- *The pot of gold:* Every child brings her own special qualities (i.e., pieces of gold) to the treatment. After participating in treatment, she will have learned many skills to deal with her bipolar disorder, which, in addition to her other positive qualities, represents the overflowing gold in the pot.

b. Recognizing Difficult Feelings (35 min.)

Activities Related to Objective

Play the "Recognizing Difficult Feelings" game:

- Using **Handout #14**, place or tape pictures of difficult feelings (i.e., Sad, Angry, Nervous, and Guilty) on each of the walls around the room.
- Have the child pick a feeling he has had, and stand by that feeling.

- Have him talk about the situation. Ask: "What caused the feeling, how did you show it, and how did you deal with it?"
- Offer other suggestions for how to deal with the difficult feeling so that the child can learn additional skills and be empowered to begin the development of problem-solving skills.
- Take a turn yourself, and model how to identify and label a feeling and think about what caused it.
- Continue to take turns standing by feelings and discussing what triggers these feelings and how we can cope with them.

Work on the "Anger Clues" worksheet (**Handout #15**). Start by explaining that when we begin to get angry, we have some type of reaction, or an anger clue. It can be in our body (clenching fists), in our feelings (crying), or in our minds or thoughts (thinking about getting into trouble).

Give the child an "Anger Clues" sheet. Have the child fill in her physiological anger clues.

Draw an analogy between losing control of anger and a volcano exploding. Anger clues are related to lava bubbling up in a volcano. No one else may be aware of the impending "explosion," but the child can sense the bubbling anger in the form of the anger clues and must use that recognition as a warning that something could be done to decrease the anger (i.e., coping skills that will be learned and practiced during the subsequent session) before her anger "explodes" out of control.

Begin the discussion of where the child feels different feelings in her body. Give the child the "Feelings are Something You Feel in Your Body" sheet (**Handout #16**) and encourage her to think of where/how she feels various emotions in her body. This is a similar procedure to the anger clues exercise, but it widens the focus to all of the emotions the child has been monitoring on her daily mood calendars.

c. Recognizing Triggers

Activities Related to Objective

Explain that now you are going to specifically focus on situations that cause the child to become angry and experience her anger clues. On a chalkboard, write "THINGS THAT BUG ME" (or the child may utilize

Handout #17: "What Are My Bugs?"). What situations cause the angry feelings?

- Ask child to share examples of things that make her angry.
- Discuss these situations and inform the child that she will generate skills to deal with these "bugs" during the next session.

4. Summary and Homework (5 min.)

Summary

Invite the parents into the session for the summary and wrap up. Ask the child to describe to her parents each of the activities she did during session and what she has learned during this session (you can help with this). Ask the parents how they did over the past week with establishing routines, helping their child identify feelings, and remaining calm during their child's anger outbursts (if there were any). Discuss and troubleshoot problems or obstacles the parents are encountering.

Homework for the Child

The child should continue to fill out the mood calendar (**Handout #9**).

Homework for the Parents

The parents should continue to work on sticking to routines, helping their child express her feelings, practice acceptance, and remain calm during anger episodes.

> ✓ *Instructions:* Remember to let the child pick a prize if she brought her mood calendars from the past two weeks. Make sure to give the Session 4 Highlights (**Handout #18**) to the parents.

I: I Can Do It!

N: No Negative Thoughts

O: Oh, How Do We Solve This Problem?

AGENDA

1. Review materials covered in last session
2. "How was your week?" Review homework
3. RAINBOW skills: problem-solving and positive thinking
   a. Positive Thinking
   b. Problem-Solving—Think and Do Skills
4. Summary and homework

Participants: Child only; check in with the parents at the end of the session

Required materials: **Handouts #9** and **#19–23**, prize basket, pen

Session length: 60 minutes

1. Review Materials Covered in the Last Session (5 min.)

Review mood and feelings spectrum, recognizing difficult feelings, and anger clues, and ask if the child has any questions.

2. How Was the Week? Review of Homework (5 min.)

Ask the child about his week. Did anything come up that he wants to discuss?

Review the child's mood calendar and discuss any problems, questions, and things that were helpful about completing it. Remind the child that he will get a prize at the end of the session for completing it.

3. RAINBOW Skills: Problem-Solving and Positive Thinking

Objective

The objective is to teach the child to cope with difficult feelings and situations by using effective problem-solving techniques and positive thinking.

Conceptual Background

Children with bipolar disorder often become so overwhelmed by their feelings that they are not able to think clearly and use good problem-solving skills. Having a concrete and systematic method for evaluating problems that arise and choosing good solutions can increase the chances that the child is able to draw upon such methods in times of distress. Therefore, a goal of these activities is to teach the child to use a clear and straightforward method of problem-solving for difficult situations that come up and the difficult emotions that ensue. In addition, as a result of years of having strong emotions, not being able to effectively cope with them, and the various consequences for conflict-ridden peer and family relationships, children with bipolar disorder often have very poor self-esteem. They feel ineffective, out of control, remorseful, and often think they are bad and unworthy. This pattern of negative thinking affects their ability to stay positive and motivated to do things better. This cycle of negative thoughts needs to be changed in order for these children to have the self-confidence and esteem to deal with difficult emotions and situations. The first step is to help them feel worthwhile. Then, they can be taught a range of skills to identify negative cognitions, reframe unhelpful thoughts into helpful ones, and use positive thinking.

a. Positive Thinking (20 min.)

Activities Related to Objective

> ✓ *Instructions: Give child the "Things That Make Me Feel Good" sheet (**Handout #19**) and "Nice Thoughts About Myself" (**Handout #20**). Help him work through each worksheet and think of positive thoughts to put in all of the bubbles. Have a discussion of the child's positive qualities, and the people, places, and activities that make him feel good.*

> ✓ *Therapist Note: Some children may have a difficult time thinking of their own positive qualities; you should be ready to supply positive characteristics of the child that you have observed during sessions.*

Discuss the importance of self-esteem in dealing with difficult feelings and situations:

- The self-esteem of the child depends on his experience with peers, teachers, and adults in his life. Have a discussion about the importance of others' reactions to him when he is experiencing difficult emotions (e.g., anger/irritability, sadness, anxiety) and how this affects his own reactions and feelings about himself.
- Help the child understand that it is important to monitor his behavior and reactions and modify his reactions in ways that lead to greater interpersonal acceptability. This will help him feel better about himself.
- Some examples of ways a child can be aware of and monitor his own reactions and responses include monitoring how he looks during the experience (e.g., show an angry, irritated expression when upset), why he is irritable (he may be sad or anxious underneath), and what it does to him in terms of others' reactions.

b. Problem-Solving—Think and Do Skills (25 min.)

Activities Related to Objective

Review the "What Are My Bugs?" worksheet (**Handout #17**, from the last session). Emphasize that in spite of the variety of "bugs" identified by the child, the one thing they all have in common is that they cause ANGER.

Review the "Anger Clues" worksheet (**Handout #15**, from the last session) and how the child's identified physiological anger clues serve as warnings that he is beginning to get angry and that he needs to try to circumvent the increasing anger via thoughts and/or actions before it is out of control (e.g., "affective storm" or "exploding volcano").

A baseball analogy and game may be used to facilitate the child's awareness of his triggers and the implementation of cognitive, behavioral, and physiological coping skills:

- Have the child place the four baseball "bases" (**Handout #21**) around the room. These bases are labeled *Mind, Body,* and *Behavior*, as well as a *Home base*. Explain that our anger clues may lead us to think, do, and feel things that make us feel MORE mad.
- Use the bases to demonstrate the connection between our feelings and cognitive, behavioral, and physiological responses. For example, when angry, we may (1) MIND base: think "I can't stand this!"; (2) BODY base: feel our fists and jaw clenching; and (3) BEHAVIOR base: yell/hit.
- But these same bases can be used to help us stay in control when we feel our anger rising, and that is when we "hit a home run." Have the child run around the bases to generate coping responses that he can do to cope with each of these angry thoughts, sensations, and actions. For example, (1) MIND base: I think "I can do this"; (2) BODY base: relax hand muscles and take deep breaths; and (3) BEHAVIOR base: walk away.
- For each BUG, the child may "run the bases" once to identify anger-increasing responses from the past, and then run the bases again to identify adaptive Mind, Body, and Behavior coping responses.

✓ *Therapist Notes:* *It may be necessary to remind the child that the goal is to generate pro-social/adaptive responses to the BUG, rather than his natural reaction, which may involve maladaptive behaviors that worsen the situation and result in undesirable consequences from authority figures (e.g., parents or teachers).*

In the event that the child suggests maladaptive behaviors, it is important to address the suggestion by discussing the undesirable resultant consequences and to brainstorm other responses that would better serve the purposes of remaining in control and dealing with the BUG adaptively.

Introduce the "Think and Do" worksheet (**Handout #22**) and explain that we will be brainstorming things that we can THINK and things that we can DO in order to stay in control when our anger clues warn us that our anger is starting to rise/bubble, before it explodes.

- Have the child pick a BUG from the "What Are My Bugs?" sheet to focus on first.
- For this problem/BUG, ask the child, "WHAT CAN I THINK?" and brainstorm with him about what he can think or say to himself to help him feel better. Write in the "Think" bubble on the "Think and Do" sheet.
- Next, ask the child, "WHAT CAN I DO?" and help brainstorm what action he could take in the particular situation in order to solve the problem/BUG. Write in the "Do" bubble on the "Think and Do" sheet.

✓ *Therapist Notes: Here, too, it may be necessary to remind the child that the goal is to generate prosocial and adaptive responses to the BUG, rather than his natural reaction, which may involve maladaptive behaviors that worsen the situation and result in undesirable consequences from authority figures (e.g., parents or teachers).*

In the event that the child suggests maladaptive behaviors, it is important to address the suggestion by discussing the undesirable consequences and to brainstorm other responses that would better serve the purposes of remaining in control and dealing with the BUG adaptively.

- After THINK and DO skills have been generated for the child's first BUG, move on to the next BUG until all have been addressed.
- At the end of the exercise, review the THINK and DO skills that were generated for the child's BUGS and why these would be good thoughts or actions to deal with the situation.

4. Summary and Homework (5 min.)

Summary

Invite the parents into the session for the summary and wrap-up. Ask the child to describe to his parents each of the activities he did and what he learned during this session. (You can help with this.) Explain the concept of Think and Do skills and how these can be useful during problem-solving for difficult situations. Explain the importance of having good self-esteem and thinking positively.

Homework for the Child

The child should continue to fill out the mood calendar (**Handout #9**); in addition, during the week, the child and parents should complete one "Think and Do" sheet (**Handout #22**) during a difficult situation.

Homework for the Parents

The parents should help their child use Think and Do skills during times of emotional distress.

✓ **Instructions:** *Remember to let the child pick a prize if he brought his mood calendars. Make sure to give the Session 5 Highlights (**Handout #23**) to the parent.*

Coping and Positive Thinking for Parents

RAINBOW INGREDIENTS

I: I Can Do It!
N: No Negative Thoughts, Live in the Now

AGENDA

1. Review materials covered in last session
2. "How was your week?" Review homework
3. RAINBOW skills:
   a. Identifying positive qualities in the child to promote and reinforce/assist the child in developing positive self-statements/coping scripts
   b. Positive self-talk
   c. Reframe negative thoughts
   d. Focus on the present; mindfulness
4. Summary and homework

Participants: Parents (or caregivers) only

Required materials: **Handouts #24–27**, pen

Session length: 90 minutes

1. Review Materials from Last Session (2 min.)

Review how the parents manage their own anger and how they model coping skills.

2. Discuss How the Week Went and Review Homework (5 min.)

How did the week go? Have the parents been working with their child to help her recognize and identify her emotions? Have they been trying new ways of interacting with the child during anger episodes, and have they developed an anger coping plan with their child? Did they have the opportunity to use it?

Did the parents have an opportunity to model appropriate coping skills during a time their child had difficulties? What coping skills did the parents model? How did the parents feel about their efforts to model coping skills? What did they find useful/not helpful? What are the long-term consequences of taking this approach with their child?

Check in with the parent about establishing routines. Have they been implementing and have they begun committing to a new routine with their child? Did they discuss specifically what is new in their routine with the child? How did the conversations go? What barriers did they encounter or foresee?

3. RAINBOW Skills

a. Identifying Positive Qualities in the Child to Promote and Reinforce (20 min.)

Objective

The objective is to help the parents promote competencies in their child by recognizing and promoting skills in their child.

Conceptual Background

Children with emotional and behavioral difficulties often struggle with self-esteem because of these difficulties. Often their problems are identified and highlighted by multiple individuals in multiple settings (e.g., peers, parents, teachers). Not surprisingly, these children may feel incompetent because of their difficulties. In addition, competencies that these children do have are often not recognized and promoted because of the tendency to be overly concerned about problematic emotions and behavior. Parents can have a major impact on helping their child recognize the competencies she has and promoting these competencies. Assisting their child in verbalizing her strengths will further increase her self-esteem. Lastly, when a child is having difficulties, her perception of herself may become distorted and negative. During these times, it will be important not only for parents to reinforce strengths and for the child to recognize her own strengths, but also for the child to have developed and to implement coping scripts (i.e., cognitive scripts children develop to balance their negative thinking about themselves and the depression they are experiencing—"I am not feeling well today but I know that I am bright, athletic, and have friends and family who care about me. The feelings I have are hard, but they will pass and I will feel better soon").

Activities Related to Objective

Discuss with the parents the concept of *competency* and the importance of identifying and promoting competencies in their child.

- What are competencies that their child has?
- Why would it be beneficial for parents to focus on competencies that their child has?

Ask the parents to make a list of their child's competencies using the "My Child's Competencies" worksheet (**Handout #24**). Then you and the parents should generate ways that the parents can promote these competencies in their child (e.g., having the parents enroll their child in activities, such as art, music, or sports, as related to the child's strengths).

You and the parents should discuss positive self-statements that parents can coach their child to say to herself. Some questions to ask the parents are:

- Why is it important to think positively about yourself?
- What are positive self-statements?
- How can we assist your child in developing positive self-statements, and how can we assist her in implementing the statements?

You and the parents should discuss coping scripts that their child can use during times of difficulty. Some items to discuss with the parents are:

- Considering that depression is cyclical for many individuals, it is likely that your child will experience a depressive episode. What can we do proactively to assist the child with managing her depression?
- One method that has been effective for children is to assist them in developing coping scripts. A coping script is a dialogue that a child can have with herself that focuses on content that helps that child cope with a situation that she knows she is likely to be involved in. What are some things that you think your child feels are strengths that she can focus on when she goes through a depressive episode? (Content can include competencies, previous experiences the child had with a depressive episode, and cognitions she feels are helpful when she is depressed.)
- How can we assist your child in developing coping scripts, and how can we assist her in implementing the scripts?

b. Positive Self-Talk (15 min.)

Objective

The objective is to help parents recognize positive experiences and use "I can do it" statements to increase their own feelings of self-efficacy.

Conceptual Background

Although negative feelings are a normal part of parenting a child with bipolar disorder, sometimes these feelings become so overwhelming that they color the way parents think about their child or their ability to manage their child's moods and behavior. Parents can be encouraged to identify positive qualities about themselves and their child, as well as to focus on positive experiences with their child. It can be helpful for parents to come up with positive self-statements such as "I can do it!" or "Today is another day" to help them through difficult situations. These thoughts may initially seem uncomfortable or unnatural, but once they become more familiar, they will offer more affirming responses to parental stress.

Activities Related to Objective

Encourage positive thinking by asking parents to come up with several positive qualities about their child. In addition, ask them to come up with positive qualities about themselves, and to identify one positive interaction they have had with their child in the past week. Explain that they can actively engage in this kind of positive thinking to help offset some of the negativity, which may often dominate their interactions with their child.

Discuss the role of positive self-statements in sustaining a more positive outlook. Suggest a few positive self-statements, and encourage parents to come up with their own "mantras" or self-statements that are relevant to them.

c. Reframe Negative Thoughts (20 min.)

Objective

The objective is to help parents recognize and reframe their own negative thoughts.

Conceptual Background

The mind becomes trained to think in negative ways—a "glass half-empty approach" to interpreting situations. These are called *cognitive distortions*, which can be corrected through retraining the mind to think in more positive ways. Parents raising a child with bipolar disorder will often have cognitive distortions (due to the stresses of parenting such a child), and the retraining will help these parents slowly convert to a more "glass half full" approach to interpreting their abilities and experiences. In addition, parents must learn to recognize the negative thoughts that they have. These are sometimes called "automatic thoughts" because they become second nature, and parents don't even recognize when they happen. Once they recognize their automatic thoughts, then they can come up with positive thoughts to replace them.

Activities Related to Objective

Explain the concept of *negative thinking* in terms of seeing the world through a negative lens (cognitive distortions) and developing "automatic thoughts." Provide examples of some of these common negative thoughts (e.g., "Nothing is ever going to make this child happy"; "This is never going to get any better"; or "I can't do this anymore"). Then, ask the parents to think about their own automatic negative thoughts.

Explain that the mind can be retrained to see the world in a different way that can have a significant impact on the parents' own moods, ability to parent, and well-being.

Pick a couple of the negative thoughts that the parents identified, and demonstrate cognitive reframing by suggesting alternative positive thoughts to replace them.

d. Focus on the Present and use Mindfulness Techniques (20 min.)

Objective

The objective is to help parents incorporate mindfulness techniques in order to stay focused on the present moment to avoid feelings of being overwhelmed and burned out.

Conceptual Background

Parents of children with bipolar disorder often feel overwhelmed and burned out in dealing with their child's emotion dysregulation and behavioral outbursts. Mindfulness can be helpful in guiding parents through stressful situations. *Mindfulness* is a technique in which a person becomes intentionally aware of his or her thoughts and actions in the present moment, non-judgmentally. Mindfulness is an activity that can be done at any time; it does not require sitting, or even focusing on breathing, but rather is done by bringing the mind to focus on what is happening in the present moment while simply noticing the mind's usual "commentary." By focusing on the present moment and staying mindful, parents may approach their child and the difficult situations that arise in a more conscious, calm, and compassionate manner.

Activities Related to Objective

Refer to resources on mindful parenting, such as those provided in **Handout #25**. Distribute **Handout #25** to the parent. Explain the concept of mindfulness and how it might be helpful.

Have the parents complete a short mindfulness exercise by shutting their eyes, focusing on their breathing, and just observing their thoughts for a few minutes using "Watching Thoughts Drift By" (**Handout #26**). Then ask the parents what it was like for them to attempt mindfulness, and explain that it is something that needs to be practiced regularly in order to see benefits.

End by going through each of the mindfulness parenting exercises, and encourage parents to try them.

4. Summary and Homework (8 min.)

Summary

Identifying and promoting competencies in children will have long-term implications for the development of their self-esteem. For parents of children with emotional and behavioral difficulties, it is very important for parents to take the lead in identifying and promoting competencies in their child. Likewise, it is important for parents to assist their child in identifying and developing positive self-statements as well as coping scripts. In addition, it is important for parents to recognize their own negative patterns of thinking and work to replace their negative thoughts with more positive and helpful ones, and stay in the present moment.

Homework for the Parents (Working with their child)

- Have the parents discuss with their child the concept of *competencies*. Parents should discuss with their child the hobbies, skills, etc., with which the child is involved. Parents should discuss with their child how she can strengthen these competencies in manageable and meaningful ways.
- Have the parents discuss the concept of positive self-statements with their child (e.g., What are the potential benefits of this approach? What are some strengths that the child should remember to think of throughout the day?)
- Have the parents discuss the use of coping scripts with their child (e.g., What are the potential benefits of a coping script? What are messages their child says to herself that she finds helpful when dealing with a depressed or angry mood?). Have the parents and child write out several coping scripts. (This can be done in a fun way like writing it out on the computer or making it into an art project.)
- Have the parents commit to practice using mindfulness techniques and mindful parenting.

✓ *Instructions: Make sure to give out the "Try at Home" sheet (**Handout #27**) for this session.*

Respectful Communication and Social Skills for Children

RAINBOW INGREDIENTS

B: Be a Good Friend

AGENDA

1. Review materials covered in last child session
2. "How was your week?" Review homework
3. RAINBOW skills: communication
   a. Nonverbal communication
   b. How to express yourself
   c. Respectful communication
   d. "I" messages
4. Summary and homework

Participants: Child only, check in with the parents at end of session

Required materials: **Handouts #9** and **#28–32**, prize basket, pen

Session length: 60 minutes

1. Review Materials Covered in the Last Child Session (5 min.)

Review problem solving, Think and Do skills, and positive thinking.

2. How Was the Week? Review Homework (5 min.)

Ask the child about his week. Did anything come up that he wants to discuss? Review the child's mood calendar and Think and Do worksheet. Remind him at the end of the session that he will get a prize for completing his homework.

3. RAINBOW Skills: Communication

Objectives

The objective is to discuss the importance of good communication, to identify respectful and disrespectful communication, and to explore different ways (verbal and nonverbal) of communicating.

Conceptual Background

For various reasons, children with bipolar disorder often have poor communication skills. Whether it is because they have missed out on important skills-building over the course of development, or because of the negative influence of mood dysregulation on their ability to communicate effectively, they can be perceived as impulsive, abrasive, bossy, and aggressive. Like most other skills, social skills can be taught and learned. Some of the important skills relevant to initiating and sustaining friendships are: calm communication, perspective-taking, empathy, and the ability to understand the impact of our behavior on others. One of the first steps in learning effective ways of communicating is to understand the role of respect, listening, and effective communication techniques.

a. Nonverbal Communication of Feelings (15 min.)

Activities Related to Objective

Begin with a discussion about nonverbal communication. Encourage the child to think of why it is important to be able to understand and communicate his feelings in a nonverbal manner. Emphasize the following points:

- Those around you can help you deal with difficult situations and feelings (e.g., when you are angry, sad, or anxious), even if you don't or can't explain it with words.

■ You can understand how others may be feeling and predict how they may act/react towards you before you engage them (e.g., recognizing that Mom is feeling angry before asking her for a privilege).

After this discussion, introduce "Feelings Charades," in which you give the child a slip of paper with a "feeling" word (e.g., *happy, sad, angry, excited*) written on it (**Handout #28**). (Don't look at the slip you give the child.) As you observe, the child must act out the feeling word on the card without speaking. You are to guess what "feeling" the child is acting out. After the correct guess, you can take a turn and the child must guess. Be sure to encourage the child and compliment him for his effort and participation.

b. Express Yourself Skills (10 min.)

Activities Related to Objective

Introduce the BEME acronym as skills that help people express themselves and communicate well with others. Ask the child to guess what each of the letters may stand for in terms of listening and communication skills—*BEME skills*: **B**ack straight; **E**ye contact; **M**outh to speak clearly; **E**ars to listen (**Handout #29**).

Model these skills in a conversation with the child; then have the child practice using those skills in a conversation with you.

> ✓ *Therapist Note: To further explain this concept, it may be helpful for you to first model the absence of BEME skills (slouched in chair, no eye contact, not speaking clearly, not paying attention to the child) and discuss how this presentation affected the child and the interaction overall. Then, you can model "correct" use of skills, and discuss with the child how the change in presentation affected the overall interaction.*

Periodically, remind the child to use his BEME skills during session and encourage him to practice these skills during the week at home and school.

c. Respectful Communication (10 min.)

Activities Related to Objective

Begin with a discussion of respect. Ask the child to define "respect" using **Handout #30.** Write down the various definitions or aspects of respect that the child generates in order to address the accuracy of each definition, and attempt to integrate them into a collectively agreed-upon definition. Emphasize the following aspects of respect:

- Being considerate
- Treating others how we want to be treated
- Being accepting and tolerant of others' rights and beliefs
- Showing kindness

Then ask the child to generate ways in which he shows respect to his parents or caretakers. Examples include:

- Being loving
- Listening
- Paying attention
- Following directions
- Not talking back

Ask the child about the results of respect (both in terms of actions or behaviors and emotions or feelings).

Follow this by asking the child to generate ways in which he shows disrespect to his parents or caretakers. Examples include:

- Swearing
- Talking back
- Having an attitude
- Interrupting
- Body language (e.g., rolling eyes, shrugging)

Follow this by asking the child about the results of disrespect (both in terms of actions or behaviors and emotions or feelings).

d. "I" Messages (10 min.)

Start this section by asking the child to guess the meaning of the term "I messages." Explain that "I" messages help the other person (e.g., parent, friend) understand how you feel and why.

Emphasize the two components of "I" messages:

- "I feel . . ."
- "Because . . . (the reason why you feel that way)."

Depending on the developmental level of the child, you can also add/say what he would like or prefer the other person to do. This will teach the child to focus on the positive, expected behavior instead of yelling and criticizing.

Normalize the struggle to contain angry feelings avoid yelling while engaging in "I" messages, as this is probably a new concept and a big change from the way the child is used to dealing with difficult situations.

Give the child examples of problem situations (e.g., "bugs" from a previous session) and have the child practice "I" messages by first completing the handout (**Handout #31**), and then acting out the scenario.

4. Summary Homework (5 min.)

Summary

Invite the parents into the session for the summary and wrap-up. Ask the child to describe to his parents each of the activities he did and what he learned during this session. (You can help with this.) Explain the concept of nonverbal communication and respectful communication and how these can be useful during social interaction and problem-solving.

Homework for the Child

The child should continue to fill out the mood calendar (**Handout #9**); in addition, the child should practice BEME skills (**Handout #29**) with the parents and at school this week.

Homework for the Parents

The parents should help remind their child to use BEME skills and "I" statements during difficult situations.

> ✓ *Instructions: Remember to let the child pick a prize if he brought his homework. Make sure to give the Session 7 Highlights (**Handout #32**) to the parents.*

Promoting Social Skills and a Balanced Life for Parents

RAINBOW INGREDIENTS

B: Be a Good Friend and Balanced Life for Parents

AGENDA

1. Review materials covered in the last parents' session
2. "How was your week?" Review homework
3. RAINBOW skill: social skills for children
   a. Promoting positive peer relationships for children
   b. Helping children problem-solve and cope effectively in challenging interpersonal situations
   c. Effective behavioral management strategies
4. RAINBOW skill: balanced life for parents
   a. Self-care
   b. Balanced life
5. Summary and homework

Participants: Parents (or caregivers) only

Required materials: **Handouts #17** and **#33–34**, pen

Session length: 90 minutes

1. Review Materials from Last Session (5 min.)

Start this session by reviewing coping skills, positive thinking, and mindfulness techniques from Session 6.

2. How Was the Week? Review Homework (5 min.)

How did the week go? Did the parents have the opportunity to discuss positive self-statements and coping scripts with their children?

3. RAINBOW Skills: Social Skills for Children

a. Promoting Positive Peer-Relationships for Children (15 min.)

Objective

The objective is to assist parents in understanding the importance of friendships for children and how to promote friendships for their child.

Conceptual Background

Peer relations are one of the most important areas of development for children. Supportive friendships are associated with decreased depression, anxiety, and loneliness for children and adolescents. Furthermore, friendship may be a buffer for children who experience difficulties in childhood. Research has shown that having even one good prosocial friendship can divert children from problems in adolescence. Friendships for children with emotional and behavioral difficulties can be difficult, however. Many children with emotional and behavioral difficulties have difficulty initiating and maintaining friendships because of their difficulties with relating to peers. They can be hypersensitive, and they may react with jealousy and bitterness in response to perceived or actual slights by their peers. Despite an intense need to be liked, children with emotional and behavioral difficulties behave in a way that pushes people away. Parents can be influential in assisting their child in developing and maintaining friendships by being able to structure play dates, sleepovers, and supervised group activities.

Activities Related to Objective

Discuss the benefits of friendships for children by asking the following questions:

- Why are friendships important for children?
- What useful skills and lessons are learned by children through the friendships they have?

Discuss difficulties the child has had in developing and maintaining friendships by asking the following:

- What have been the difficulties your child has had in developing and maintaining friendships? Why?

Ask the parents about peer settings in which their child feels competent in her social skills. Have the parents discuss ways of increasing these types of opportunities for their child. Parents should also be prompted to identify new situations where their child can interact with her friends to promote these relationships (e.g., sleepovers, play dates, and supervised group activities). How can the parents increase the frequency of these activities?

b. Promoting Coping and Problem-Solving Around Difficult Situations (20 min.)

Objective

The objective is to assist parents in helping their child use effective communication strategies for navigating through difficult situations before they escalate.

Conceptual Background

Difficult or distressing situations happen. The key to managing these situations is to minimize the child's emotional or behavioral disturbances associated with these stressful events. Effective communication between children and caregivers can "head off" escalating emotions and behavior in multiple ways. During a calm period free from distraction, parents can encourage their child to identify which situations represent the "bugs" that quickly lead to escalation, and to share any thoughts or feelings related to these events. By using active listening skills, parents can help their child feel understood and supported; additionally, through the use of "I" statements, parents can communicate their own thoughts and feelings about stressful situations in a way that minimizes negative interactions. Through effective communication, parents and child alike may voice respect for each other, and develop a greater sense of teamwork when coping with difficult situations.

Additionally, parents can use effective communication strategies to help their child limit behavioral and emotional escalation the next time a "bug" rears its head. As an example, through practice sessions, parents may help their child communicate appropriate expressions of frustration before it intensifies. Parents can then respond to these "signals" by clearly reflecting the emotion and then proactively assisting their child to minimize escalation. Finally, when parents and their child successfully divert an emotional or behavioral disruption, they can communicate their happiness with each other as they celebrate this accomplishment together!

Activities Related to Objective

Discuss the triggers for emotional and behavioral escalation. Which triggers seem to occur most frequently? What behaviors are the most difficult to control?

Discuss problems the child has had in managing difficult situations. Ask the parents to describe how their child typically communicates feelings of distress. What interactions or interventions have the parents found *not* helpful once the escalation starts?

Ask the parents about their own thoughts and feelings during these situations. Then parents can reflect upon thoughts that are most effective in helping them manage difficult situations and contain their child's emotional and behavioral escalation once it starts.

Discuss ways of building teamwork when working with the child to problem-solve difficult situations. These include discussing their child's "bugs" with the child during calm periods, using active listening skills in order to help their child feel understood, sharing their own thoughts or feelings through "I" statements, and setting a collaborative, nonjudgmental tone when discussing difficult situations.

Identify ways to help the child plan and practice appropriate coping strategies for managing difficult situations. These include helping the child recognize triggers through the use of the "What Are My Bugs?" sheet (**Handout #17**); generating and evaluating a range of possible thoughts, behavioral responses, and outcomes associated with a difficult situation; and role playing. Help the child develop prosocial or adaptive responses, as opposed to natural reactions that may result in maladaptive behaviors and negative consequences.

c. Behavioral Management (20 min.)

Objective

The objective is to assist parents in managing their child's behavioral escalation once it occurs.

Conceptual Background

At times, there may be no way of avoiding periods of emotional escalation. On these occasions, it is important to remember that it is nobody's fault—caregivers did not cause the escalation, and a child with an emotional and behavioral disturbance often cannot control these rages once they start. During these situations, caregivers can practice strategies to contain emotional or behavioral disturbance. Parents can be influential in modeling appropriate responses to difficult situations in the moment; then, *afterward*, caregivers and the child can review the situation and problem-solve ways of managing similar situations in the future. The overall goal is to maximize opportunities for working together, and minimize the time working against each other.

Activities Related to Objective

Discuss management of emotional or behavioral escalation after it starts. It is important to disengage from any interactions that serve to further escalate the disturbance. Of course, the safety of person and property is foremost, and you can discuss with the parents how they can effectively contain escalation through the use of a "safe zone" or other environmental manipulation to provide a safe place for the child until calm.

Help the parents consider appropriate consequences for behavioral escalation. This will probably *not* be helpful if addressed *during* a period of acute distress; however, inclusion of the child when developing appropriate consequences, and restitution after the child has calmed, can limit adversarial interactions and even help the child to feel like an active participant when reestablishing stability. It can be an empowering message to suggest that, although the child may not be able to control her rages, she can ultimately feel a sense of maturity by responsibly addressing rule transgressions.

Discuss self-soothing activities the child has effectively engaged in previously, or may benefit from, to use during escalation. Generate a list of soothing activities and places that can be used, with close supervision, to help the child safely calm down (e.g., punching a pillow, holding an ice cube, taking a warm bath).

4. RAINBOW Skill: Living a Balanced Life

a. Promoting Parental Self-Care (10 min.)

Objective

The objective is to maximize opportunities for self-care so that parents may more effectively manage the home environment, utilize coping strategies during stressful situations, and consistently assist their child with practicing helpful coping strategies.

Conceptual Background

Balancing all of life's demands, including managing a busy household, attending to life responsibilities, and coping with the ups and downs of a child's bipolar disorder, takes significant time, energy, and effort. These demands are often both physically and emotionally exhausting. In order for parents to help their child practice self-care and coping skills during stressful situations, it is important for parents to engage in their own self-care. Just as a high-performance car requires fuel and routine maintenance to run, or a garden requires nutrients and a consistent water source to bloom, parents need to ensure greatest possible health and strength for themselves to both meet the demands of a high-octane life, and nourish a flourishing home environment.

Sometimes parents or caregivers are reluctant to engage in self-care, or they think that their own self-care is relatively unimportant. They may feel guilty about taking time for themselves, or become used to sacrificing their own time for the sake of the family. It is important to recognize that *engaging in self-care is not selfish*. Self-care is about developing, or further increasing, parents' reserves of strength so that they can be there for their child when their child needs them most!

Activities Related to Objective

Discuss examples of how coping skills are utilized most effectively during periods of relative health and replenishment, and how people tend to fall back on less effective strategies when fatigued or experiencing a period of diminished health.

Instruct the parents to reflect upon a personal health inventory. Ask them to:

- Evaluate current areas of their personal health, including physical, emotional, spiritual, life, and recreation aspects.
- Discuss enjoyable activities they engage in (or would engage in if they had the time) that are uniquely their own. Which enjoyable activities involve (or would involve) the family together? (Either way, the focus is on activities that provide refreshment.)

Discuss how each aspect of personal health interlocks with other areas, such that as one component of health improves, others may also improve. Have parents identify ways of improving self-care in one or more areas of health this week, no matter how small (e.g., taking time to eat breakfast, scheduling a brisk 10-minute walk at the park, calling a friend on the phone).

Help parents identify barriers to self-care, and problem-solve ways to improve self-care over the next week. This may include asking adult family members or friends for assistance in order to free up time for healthy activities.

It is important for parents to be wary of negative thoughts or judgmental self-statements as they plan for self-care activities. Parents can identify these thoughts during the session, and then use their reframing skills to create more accurate thoughts about taking time for themselves. Ultimately, when parents feel healthier, they may also feel more prepared to manage life demands, including their child's physical and mental health!

b. Finding Balance (10 min.)

Objective

The objective is to help parents recognize the importance of a balanced approach to their own lives; to help parents take account of their lifestyles and ways they can live more balanced lifestyles.

Conceptual Background

There is truth to the cliché that "you can't help anybody else until you help yourself." Along these lines, a happier person makes for a more effective person. Therefore, it is essential that parents take care of their own needs and create a sense of well-being through actively engaging in pleasurable activities and nurturing their adult relationships. Parents may feel guilty about taking time away from their child, especially an ill child, but it should be emphasized that this is an important part of their child's treatment and recovery. Children look to their parents for examples of how to live and how to form relationships; contented and fulfilled parents provide excellent role models! Parents will also be better able to weather storms and difficult situations if they themselves are rested and well.

Activities Related to Objective

Discuss the concept of taking care of oneself and why it is important, in particular, when parenting a child with bipolar disorder.

Ask the parents to identify things they currently do to take care of themselves. Ask them to also think about activities that they enjoy, but that they do not do enough of and would like to incorporate into their routines. Brainstorm ways to incorporate these activities into their daily lives. Explain this as taking time to "recharge your batteries." Explain the concept of "carving out pieces of your own pie."

Using the Balanced Lifestyle sheet (**Handout #33**), ask the parents to identify what percentage of time they spend doing various activities in their lives, including work, taking care of kids, pleasurable activities, and relaxation ("real" pie chart). Then on the "ideal" pie chart, help the parents redistribute the percentages so that they feel they have adequate time devoted to self-care activities. Discuss how the parents can begin to incorporate these activities to balance out their lives through increasing self-care activities on their pie chart.

Discuss the importance of adult relationships and the nurturance of friendships and romantic relationships. You and the parents can brainstorm ways of incorporating time for important relationships.

5. Summary and Homework (5 min.)

Summary

Summarize the themes from today's session:

- Understanding and developing positive peer relationships for their child and promoting these relationships in their child
- Helping the child cope with difficult interpersonal situations

- Effective behavioral management
- Promoting self-care and developing a more balanced lifestyle for the parents

Ask the parents if they have any questions.

Review the parents' understanding of triggers, appropriate vs. inappropriate approaches to problem-solving, using effective communication strategies, and timing of interventions.

Homework for the Parents (Working with their Child)

- Have the parents talk to their child about setting up a peer-related, structured activity.
- Ask parents to talk to their child about her "bugs."
- The parents should strategize a plan to cope with difficult situations, both when triggers are identified/anticipated (i.e., practice "Think and Do"), and after stressful situations develop (disengagement, containment).
- Have the parents and child develop appropriate consequences that empower their child to perceive a sense of responsibility for making a positive impact following an outburst.
- Instruct the parents to complete **Handout #33** on developing a more balanced lifestyle.

> ✓ *Instructions: Make sure to give out the "Try at Home" sheet (**Handout #34**) for this session.*

SESSION #9   Family Problem Solving

O: Oh, How Do We Solve This Problem?

AGENDA

1. Review materials covered in the last session
2. "How was your week?" Review homework
3. RAINBOW skill: family coping and problem solving
4. Summary and homework

Participants: Parents, child, siblings

Required materials: **Handout #35**, prize basket, pen

Session length: 60 minutes

1. Review Materials from Last Session (2 min.)

Review promoting positive social relationships, behavioral management and coping strategies, and living a balanced life.

2. How Was the Week? Review Homework (8 min.)

Did the parents identify new situations in which their child can interact with his friends to promote positive relationships (e.g., sleepovers, play dates, and supervised group activities)? What were the difficulties? How did the child respond to these opportunities?

Did the parents create a balance pie chart, goals, and schedules? Were the parents able to find time for self-care? If not, what got in the way? If the parents were able to attain more balanced lifestyles this week, how did it feel? What did the parents learn from practicing more balanced lifestyles?

Did the parents work with the child to identify and discuss difficult situations that trigger emotional and behavioral difficulties? Did the child and parents find a "quiet" time to talk about triggers in a way that felt like they were working as a team to problem-solve together? What were the difficulties identified together? Did the parents utilize active listening skills and "I" statements? How did the child respond?

Did the parents help the child develop a list of possible prosocial and adaptive responses to challenging situations? What were the difficulties encountered when conducting this exercise?

Did the parents disengage from interaction during behavioral or emotional escalation? Did the parents help the child contain affective storms? If not, what got in the way? Looking back now, what was (or would have been) helpful for managing the situation? Did behavioral consequences provide opportunities for the child to reflect on the positive aspect of making amends?

3. RAINBOW Skills: Family Coping and Problem Solving (40 min.)

Objective

The objective is to improve family interactions by helping families navigate difficult situations, minimize behavioral escalation once it occurs, and foster affiliation among family members through emphasizing shared experiences, positive feelings, and common goals.

Conceptual Background

The previous session focused on helping children with behavioral or emotional difficulties manage stressful situations. Often, behavioral and emotional escalation disrupts family activities, and it can negatively affect interactions among family members. This session broadens the scope of intervention to help the entire family manage difficult situations in order to limit family conflict and improve familial interactions.

Activities Related to Objective

Discuss with the parents, child, and siblings any patterns in which behavioral escalation may influence negative thoughts and feelings among family members, which then may lead to increased conflict between family members.

- Identify how each family member experiences episodes.
- How do family members express their feelings associated with episodes? What makes it difficult for family members to communicate uncomfortable feelings with each other?
- What types of family interactions or interventions have family members found to be *not* helpful during an episode of behavioral or emotional disturbance?

Discuss ways of helping the family identify thoughts and express feelings with each other in ways that promote positive coping and limit additional conflict. Emphasize that it is important for all family members to have opportunities to talk about their experiences and to have that experience respected by the family. It is also important for all family members to understand that in many situations, children with bipolar disorder cannot control their behaviors once they escalate. It is nobody's fault, and these episodes do not typically reflect how the child actually feels about family members.

Discuss ways of helping the child and other family members to problem-solve difficult situations: these include discussing "bugs" together during calm periods, using active listening skills, using "I" statements, and fostering a respectful, nonjudgmental environment for each family member to feel understood.

Help family members identify how to plan and practice appropriate coping strategies for managing difficult situations: these include helping the child recognize triggers through the use of the "What Are My Bugs?" sheet; generating and evaluating a range of possible thoughts, behavioral responses, and outcomes associated with a difficult situation; and role playing.

Discuss how the family can develop a plan for working as a team to manage emotional or behavioral escalation after it starts. For example, parents can disengage from any interactions that serve to further escalate the disturbance; siblings can immediately move to another room and begin an enjoyable activity.

Finally, help the family focus on the positive interactions of family members, and find ways of highlighting or celebrating positive experiences as they occur. Reinforcement of adaptive, inclusive, and helpful interactions (e.g., when siblings relate positively with each other, or alternatively, when siblings respond in an adaptive fashion to a stressful or escalating situation) is likely to result in repetition of the positive behaviors in the future.

4. Summary and Homework (10 min.)

Summary

Summarize the themes from today's session:

- Ensuring all family members feel respected
- Developing family-wide strategies for problem solving and coping with difficult situations
- Reinforcing positive interactions among family members

Homework for the Family

- Include all family members in a discussion about their "bugs."
- Strategize a family plan to cope with difficult situations, both when triggers are identified/anticipated (i.e., practice "Think and Do"), and after stressful situations develop (disengagement, containment).
- Have family members role-play multiple possible responses to a stressful situation, and then choose the response that is likely to result in the best outcome (i.e., "act out" the "Think and Do" worksheet).
- Encourage the child to continue to complete the mood calendar.

> ✓ *Instructions: Remember to let the child pick a prize if he brought his mood calendars from the past two weeks. Make sure to give out the "Try at Home" handout (**Handout #35**) for this session.*

Creating Pleasant Memories
and Finding Support

RAINBOW INGREDIENTS

W: Ways to Find Social Support

AGENDA

1. Review materials covered in last session
2. "How was your week?" Review homework
3. RAINBOW skills: finding social support
   a. Social support for parents
   b. Social support for children
   c. Support Tree activity
4. Summary and homework

Participants: Parents and child

Required materials: **Handouts #36–37**, markers, pencils, or crayons

Session length: 60 minutes

1. Review Materials Covered in the Last Session (5 min.)

Review the concepts of respect, family coping and problem-solving, and the importance of positive family interactions.

2. How Was the Week? Review Homework and Concepts of Family Coping and Problem-Solving Around Affective Storms (5 min.)

Did the family share their "bugs" in a way that did not place blame on other family members (i.e., did the family members use "I" statements)? Did other family members use effective listening skills in a way that helped each family member feel understood and supported when sharing "bugs"? What were some of the common themes shared by all family members?

Did the family develop a list of possible prosocial and adaptive responses to challenging situations? Did this discussion occur in a way that felt like everyone was included as a team to problem-solve together? How did the role-playing and practice exercises go? How did family members enact the plan over the course of the week? What were the difficulties?

Did the family identify and reinforce positive interactions and adaptive responses to stressful situations? How did it feel to reflect on the positive aspects of family life? Did this change the way family members think about each other and stressful events?

3. RAINBOW Skills: Finding Social Support

Objectives

The objectives are to maximize opportunities for social support in order to improve parental health and well-being so that parents may feel more energized to manage stressful situations, help their child utilize effective coping strategies for limiting emotional or behavioral outbursts, and help their child develop his own social skills; to help the child understand the importance of having good social supports and reaching out to others for help when he is in need; to help parents and child together identify important individuals in their social support network as well as to create a visual reminder of supportive others to use in times of need.

Conceptual Background

Looking back through history, even the best generals did not fight their battles alone. Regardless of their resources, they made sure to surround themselves with support, including reserves that could be called upon if needed, and important individuals in whom to confide and with whom to strategize.

A significant aspect of self-care is the establishment and maintenance of friendships or other social contacts. Social interactions are pleasurable in themselves, which improves our well-being and self-confidence to handle tough situations.

Social support can be called upon to assist with multitasking or open up time for other self-care behaviors. Additionally, parents can rely on social support for validation.

During the tough times, it can be encouraging for parents to feel that they are not alone, and during the good times, it can be exciting to celebrate with others!

Finally, as parents develop their own social support, they are modeling healthy coping mechanisms for their child; parents can then assist the child to develop and maintain his own social support system.

a. Promoting Social Support in Parents (15 min.)

Activities Related to Objective

Work with the parents to focus on the "layers" of their social support system. To begin, ask the parents to identify the select few people to whom they can honestly express themselves and with whom they can share experiences (both the difficult times and the celebrations). These are the people who help parents feel best about themselves (i.e., their "core support" group).

Parents then identify "go to" people inside or outside the family who might assist the parents with enacting their plans for self-care, either through shared participation in a healthy activity (e.g., a walking partner), or through occasional help with multitasking in order to open up time for self-care (e.g., picking up a child from school to allow for 20 minutes of meditation, or taking the child to the park to allow a parent's lunch visit with a friend). These may or may not be the same members of their "core support" group.

Parents then discuss their interests, and develop ways of developing social connections with others related to these enjoyable activities (even if it is for a limited time once per month or so). Social activities may include: shopping, going to the gym, going out to lunch with a group, fishing, participating in religious organization activities, or going to a ballgame. Parents develop a plan for trying out at least one of these activities with someone else over the next week.

You and the parents then discuss and evaluate methods of widening and utilizing social support networks, as well as strategies to work through barriers to increasing social contacts.

It is important for the parents to be wary of negative thoughts or judgmental self-statements related to social support. Parents can identify these negative thoughts during this session, and then use their reframing skills to create more accurate thoughts about developing and utilizing their social support contacts.

All of the foregoing activities help the parents develop methods for helping their child utilize and increase social support networks. Additionally, problem-solve with the parents around potential barriers to social support for their child.

b. Social Support for Children (15 min.)

Activities Related to Objective

Role-play a scenario about seeking help. Begin by asking the child the ways in which he can communicate the need for help from those around him. Make sure that the following points are emphasized:

- Try not to interrupt the other person.
- Ask politely for help rather than demanding it.
- Try to be patient if help cannot be given immediately.
- Try to limit help-seeking behavior to only when it is needed.

Discuss the activity of seeking help from others as a strength or skill rather than as a weakness or a feeling of dependence. Ask about times when the child needed help in his life (and how he went about seeking help) and ask him to think about strong people in his life and how they might have needed (or will need) help in their own lives.

Next, you and the parents take turns pairing up with the child and create and role-play help-seeking scenarios. These may include role playing as a parent–child dyad, teacher–student dyad, or friend–friend dyad.

Encourage the child to offer feedback in terms of how it felt for him to seek help and how it felt when he was approached for help. You may coach or offer feedback and reinforce his efforts.

c. Support Tree Activity (15 min.)

Activities Related to Objective

Give the parents and child their individual copies of the "Support Tree" drawing (**Handout #36**) and encourage them to identify and discuss special people in their lives whom they feel they can count on for support. These individuals are the special people in their lives who may help them recover from depression or rage attacks, whom they can rely on; whom they can play with, go out with, talk to, have fun with, just be there for them; who'll listen to them, and who provide some form of comfort. These individuals may be family members, friends, teachers, therapists, neighbors, other role models, or even pets.

Instruct the child and parents to list the names of these individuals on the "Support Tree" drawing in any order they like (e.g., some people place the most important individuals at the base, some place them at the top, whereas others have no ordering or ranking system) and then to color the drawing.

Discuss how at times it may feel like nobody is there for support, especially when one is feeling lonely and depressed. Those are the times when it is most important or encouraging to reflect on the "Support Tree."

Ask the child and parents to discuss their "Support Tree" and praise them for their contribution.

4. Summary and Homework (5 min.)

Summary

Summarize the themes from today's session:

- Developing and maintaining a plan for increasing social support
- Helping child practice seeking social support

Homework for the Parents

- Have the parents try at least one new or additional socially related activity.

- Each parent should take the time to share his or her thoughts and feelings with a member of a core support group, either in person or via phone.
- The parents should assist the child with developing and maintaining social support contacts through completion of "Support Tree" activities and "Think and Do" worksheets.

Homework for the Child

- The child should keep practicing his "Think and Do Skills" (**Handout #22**) and request help from the family, too.
- The child should also continue to fill out the mood calendar (**Handout #9**).

✓ **Instructions:** *Remember to let the child pick a prize if he brought his mood calendars from the past week. Make sure to give out the "Try at Home" sheet (**Handout #37**) for this session.*

Reflecting on RAINBOW Experience and Tools Learned

1. Review materials covered in last session
2. "How was your week?" Review homework
3. RAINBOW binder and review
4. Review of skills with parents
5. Summary and wrap-up

Participants: Child only (parents/caregivers for second half)

Required materials: RAINBOW binder; three copies of **Handout #1**; **Handout #13**; **Handout #38**; construction paper for RAINBOW binder covers

Session length: 60 minutes

1. Review Materials Covered in the Last Session (5 min.)

The topics for review include the importance of identifying and using social support networks and encouraging the child to request social support.

2. How Was the Week? Review Homework (5 min.)

Did the child think of more people to add to her support tree? Did she reach out to anyone for support over the past week?

3. RAINBOW Binder (20 min.)

The purpose of this activity is for the child and you to work together to compile the RAINBOW notebook, and by doing so, to review all the various lessons and strategies that were learned.

Ask the child to choose two sheets of construction paper from a selection of colors for the back and the front covers of her binder. Staple the "RAINBOW" picture (**Handout #13**) to the front of the construction paper cover. The first four pages to be put in the book are: (1) the Owner page; (2) the Skills Learned page; (3) the Favorite Activity page; and (4) the Positive Family Change page (**Handout #38**). Then the rest of the prior activity sheets are added in the order in which they were completed.

Help the child recall examples of skills learned, her favorite activity, and positive changes that have occurred in her family. Follow this by discussing all of the skills and tools learned over the course of the therapy and how this book can be used as a reminder.

4. Review of Basic Concepts and Skills (parents come in for this part) (25 min.)

Objective

The objective is to review the general concepts of RAINBOW; to discuss the child's and parents' perspectives of their skill development for managing difficult situations, as well as the parents' observations of skill development in their child.

Conceptual Background

Over the past eleven weeks, the child and parents have learned about the basic components of RAINBOW and have practiced strategies for coping more effectively with pediatric bipolar disorder. Children and families now have additional skills for establishing healthy routines, managing difficult situations, improving communication, enhancing overall coping through changed thinking patterns, and building social support systems. This session provides the family with the opportunity to reflect upon the development of particular RAINBOW skills and to identify ways that they can continue to practice RAINBOW skills after completing the therapy.

Activities Related to Objective

The parents, child, and you discuss each component of RAINBOW (**Handout #1**, three copies) and how they fit together. The parents and child share which RAINBOW skills have developed most over the course of the therapy, and they talk about which skills have been most helpful to them and their families. The parents and child also identify which RAINBOW skills have been most difficult to apply consistently, and you work with the parents to formulate a plan for managing residual barriers.

The parents and child reflect on specific instances when they were able to practice RAINBOW skills to successfully manage stressful situations. Finally, the parents and child discuss how they plan to continue developing RAINBOW skills after completion of the sessions.

5. Summary and Wrap-up (5 min.)

Ask the child to share her RAINBOW book with her parents. You, the child, and the parents can go through the book together and talk about all of the skills and tools learned, and how these must continue to be practiced.

Discuss that next week will be the last session in this phase of treatment.

> ✓ *Instructions: Remember to let child pick a prize if she brought her mood calendars from the past week.*

AGENDA

1. Reflecting on the therapy experience
2. Positive qualities activity: Highlight each other's strengths and positive qualities
3. Discuss follow-up/maintenance plan
4. Summary and wrap-up

Participants: Child and parents/caregivers

Required materials: None

Session length: 60 minutes

1. Reflecting on the Therapy Experience (30 min.)

Objective

The objective is to share the thoughts and feelings associated with participating in the RAINBOW program.

Conceptual Background

Participation in the RAINBOW program requires a significant time commitment, both to attend sessions and to consistently complete homework assignments during the week. Over the course of the program, children and parents try strategies that are possibly both unfamiliar and uncomfortable at first. Additionally, participation in therapy challenges each child and parent to share thoughts and feelings with one another and with the therapist, and to honestly reflect upon thoughts and feelings within themselves. Over time, however, parents and the child alike have persistently developed new skills, as well as new ways of relating to one another in order to cope more effectively with bipolar disorder.

This is a time to reflect back on all of those instances when the child or parent discovered a reserve of strength in themselves, their child, and their families. It is a time to talk about what worked and what did not work as well. And, just as important, it is a time to reflect upon the strengthening of their relationships and the family's commitment to managing this disorder.

Activities Related to Objective

- This is the time for the parents and you to recognize and celebrate the effort demonstrated by the child each week.
- Ask the parents to reflect back to their initial thoughts and feelings related to their participation in the therapy.
- Discuss the parents' initial hopes associated with participating in the therapy. Which aspects of the therapy turned out to be the most beneficial?
- Talk about any initial skepticism the parents had related to starting the therapy. Reflecting back now, what was the source of these doubts? Did participation in the therapy ease these concerns as it progressed? If so, what elements of the therapy helped more than expected?
- Did the parents find themselves more comfortable sharing thoughts and feelings as time went on? Did the child feel more comfortable reflecting upon difficult topics?
- Ask the parents to identify how they managed barriers over the course of the RAINBOW program. In what ways did the family members help each other work through difficult circumstances?
- What aspects of this therapy were most effective in helping the parents feel more supported and better able to manage difficult situations? Were there aspects of the therapy that were less helpful? How would parents characterize their therapy experience overall?

■ Ask the child:

    ■ What things have you learned in therapy?

    ■ What has changed in your family over the past 12 weeks?

    ■ What would you like to have done in therapy that we didn't do?

2. Positive Qualities Activity (10 min.)

Provide an opportunity for the child to receive positive feedback from both you and the parents. Have the parents highlight positive qualities about their child that they have noticed over the course of the therapy. In turn, have the child talk about positive qualities in his parents that he has noticed over the course of therapy.

3. Discuss Follow-up and Maintenance Plan (10 min.)

This is a broad discussion on the vision, plans of follow-up care, support networks that the family belongs to, and connection to existing treatment agencies. This will ensure that they leave with a sense of hope and connection to go back to, as they disperse.

4. Summary and Wrap-up (10 min.)

Summarize the themes of today's session: reflect on participation in the RAINBOW therapy and on the development of applicable skills to enhance coping with pediatric bipolar disorder.

Talk about the next steps. Will the family come in for maintenance therapy? Will they continue with another therapist?

Say goodbyes!

Handouts

Accessing Programs *ThatWork* Forms and Worksheets Online

All forms and worksheets from books in the Programs *ThatWork* (PTW) series are made available digitally shortly following print publication. You may download, print, save, and digitally complete them as PDF files. To access the forms and worksheets, please visit http://www.oup.com/us/ttw.

RAINBOW

R outine

A ffect Regulation

I can do it

N o negative thoughts & live in the Now

B e a good friend & Balanced lifestyle for parents

O h, how can we solve this problem?

W ays to get support

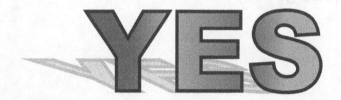

NO

NOT SURE

Why Am I Here? Question Sheet

Ask child the questions below. Follow up with questions that draw out each set of responses. Address any misunderstandings.

Do you know why you are here?
(Follow up – Why do you think you're here? Who told you?)

Have you been to a clinic or seen a counselor before?
(Follow up – What was it like? What did you think it would be like?)

Have you ever been in a group with other kids or families before?
(Follow up – What kind of group? What was it like? What did you like about it? What didn't you like about it?)

Do you think that you are here because you are in trouble?
(Follow up – Why do you think you are here? Who told you that?)

Do you think that you are here because you are bad?
(Follow up – Why do you think you are here? Who told you that?)

Do you think that this is going to be fun?
(Follow up – Why not? We're going to make it as much fun as we can!)

Getting to Know You

1. What do you like to do for fun?

_____

2. Do you have any pets?

_____

3. What do you do well?

_____

4. Where are you from?

_____

5. What is your favorite subject in school?

_____

6. Who are the important people in your life?

_____

7. What is your favorite food?

_____

8. Where would you like to go for vacation?

_____

9. What is your favorite sport?

_____

10. What color do you like most?

_____

Feelings poster

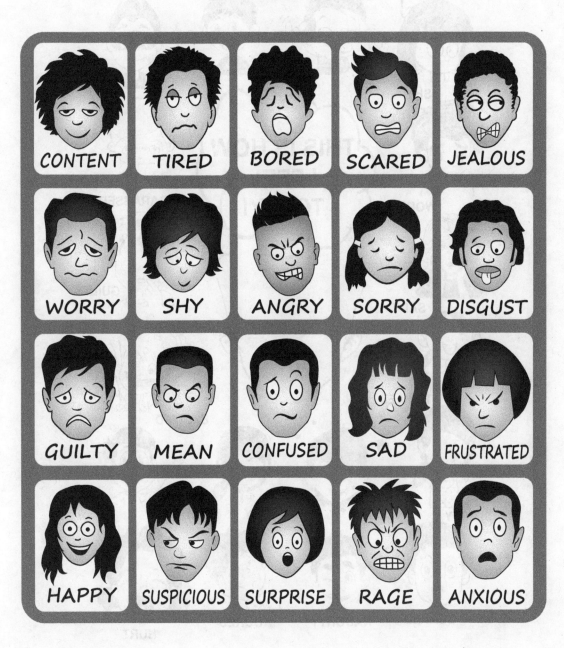

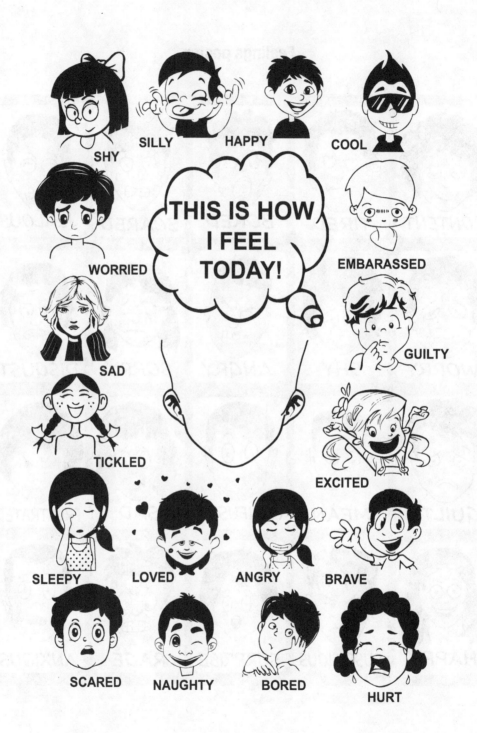

My Feeling Today Is...

Name:_____   Date:_____

Directions: Draw in the expression that best describes your current feeling

| HAPPY | SAD | ANGRY | AFRAID |

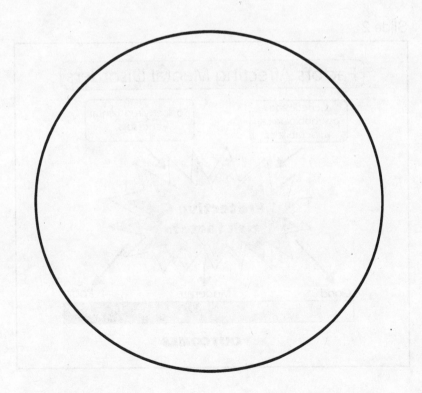

RAINBOW Psychoeducation

Slide 1

RAINBOW
Psychoeducation

What is Pediatric Bipolar Disorder?

Slide 2

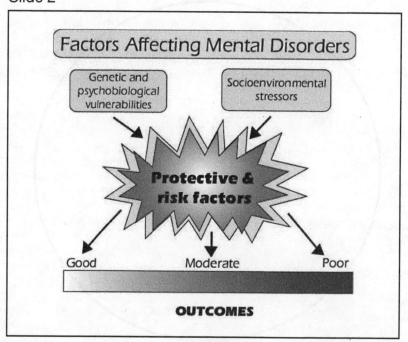

Slide 3

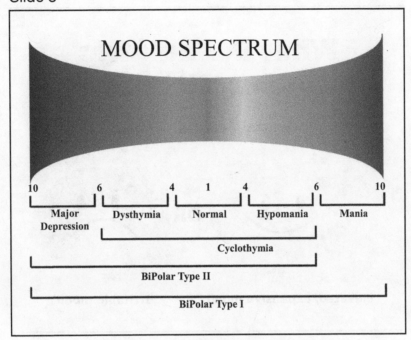

MOOD SPECTRUM

| 10 | 6 | 4 | 1 | 4 | 6 | 10 |

Major Depression   Dysthymia   Normal   Hypomania   Mania

Cyclothymia

BiPolar Type II

BiPolar Type I

Slide 4

What is Pediatric Bipolar Disorder?

An Overview

- **Mood disorder with episodes of mania, depression, or mixed (elements of both), and associated symptoms**
  - **Bipolar Spectrum: Type I, II, Unspecified subtypes**
  - **Severity, duration of episodes → diagnosis**
- **"Brain" disorder**
- **Pediatric bipolar disorder has unique features compared to adult-onset**

Slide 5

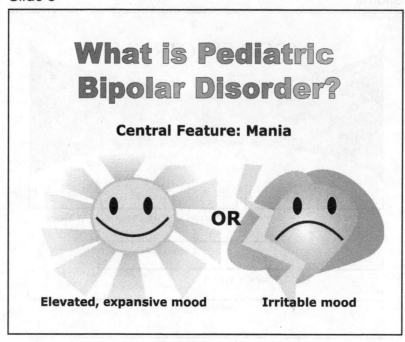

What is Pediatric Bipolar Disorder?

Central Feature: Mania

OR

Elevated, expansive mood   **Irritable mood**

Slide 6

Core Features of Bipolar Disorder

Mood: elevated, expansive or irritable

Elevated/Expansive Mood	Irritable Mood
• Excited	• Constantly irritable
• Giggly, laughing fits	• Aggressive
• Silly	• Hard to transition
• Giddy	• Abrasive
• Grandiose	• Hostile in words
• Constantly on the go	• Kicking, screaming
• Joking and feeling invincible	• Intense & inconsolable tantrums; "rage episodes"
• Overwhelming, inappropriate for setting	• Out of proportion to the psychosocial stresses around them

Slide 7

Inflated self-esteem
or grandiosity

Symptoms:
**Uncritical self-confidence; unrealistic, grandiose
beliefs about one's abilities or powers**

Examples:
- **"I am the best baseball player in America."**
- **"I will teach the teachers how to run the school.
  They don't know what they are doing."**
- **"I am absolutely sure that I will get an Oscar
  before I am 35."**
- **"I am going to make millions. I don't need to go to
  school."**

   (all with no good evidence)

Slide 8

Decreased need for sleep

Symptoms:
**Not sleeping a lot, but still feeling extremely energetic;
getting a few hours of sleep a night, but not tired**

Examples:
- **A five year old will spend hours playing in their
  room, full of energy, getting up from the bed, or
  never going to bed, singing at 2 AM, or watching TV,
  and does not feel tired in the morning**
- **10 year old makes food in the middle of the night, is
  noisy, and walks around**
- **" I feel like an energizer bunny."**

Slide 9

Pressure to keep talking

Symptoms:

Loud, rapid and difficult to interrupt speech; non-stop talking; talking so fast that it's difficult to keep up; changes topics quickly

Examples:

- Constantly talking & not letting others have a say
- Appearing dominating or anxious or continually seeking attention
- Excessive speech is couched as entertainment for others

Slide 10

Flight of ideas or racing thoughts

Symptoms:

Jumping from one idea to another; feeling like thoughts are moving really fast

Examples:

- Feeling like thoughts are on "fast forward" or "overdrive"
- Lack of control over thoughts

Slide 11

Constant goal directed activity

Symptoms:
Excessively plans and/or pursues a goal

Examples:
- " I ran for a class president, I lost it. But I am fund raising for One Direction."
- "He feeds the dog, wants to play chess, do art, fight with brothers & sisters all in one hour."

Slide 12

Distractibility

Symptoms:
Attention easily diverted to irrelevant or unimportant things; attention shifts from one thing to another

Examples:
- Can't accomplish homework because of something on TV
- Their focus moves from a game, to something on TV, to noises outside

Slide 13

Excessive involvement in pleasurable activities (poor judgment & risk taking)

Symptoms:
Reckless behavior without thinking of consequences; impaired judgment and impulsivity

Examples:
- **Excessive interest in or discussion of sexual activity**
- **Inappropriate attire**
- **Looking at inappropriate content (magazines, web sites, chat lines)**
- **Excessive self-stimulation or exposure of private parts**
- **Inappropriate play with others**
- **Use of parents credit cards or constantly pressuring parents to buy expensive things**

Slide 14

Signs of Depression

Typical Signs
- **Appears sad and tearful**
- **Does not enjoy playing, friendships, TV**
- **Not eating, picky with food**
- **Unable to sleep**
- **Slowed down/restless**
- **Unable to concentrate on homework**
- **Grades are falling**
- **Avoids school**

Associated Symptoms
- **Clingy**
- **Disrespectful of authority**
- **Crying easily**
- **More sensitive to rejection**
- **Poor frustration tolerance**
- **Withdrawn**
- **Fearful**
- **Separation anxiety**
- **Somatic symptoms**
- **Suicidal thoughts**

Slide 15

The Role of the Brain in Pediatric Bipolar Disorder

Neurobiological Underpinnings

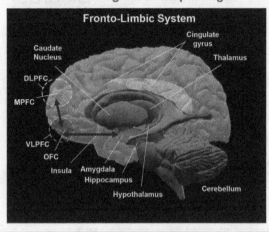

Slide 16

Unique Characteristics of Pediatric Bipolar Disorder

- **Extreme mood lability or mood dysregulation**
  - **Significant irritability or "rage episodes"**
  - **Mixed mood states: mania and depression**
- **Rapid cycling between mood states (>1/day)**
- **Comorbid disorders (ADHD, ODD, Anxiety)**

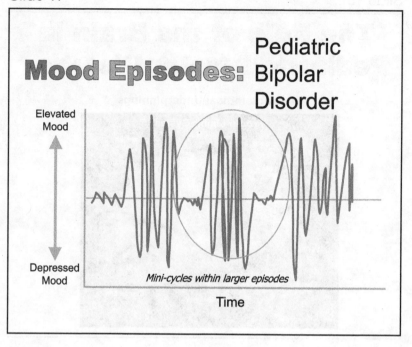

Common Comorbid Disorders

- **Attention Deficit Hyperactivity Disorder**
  - Symptoms: doesn't listen/follow instructions, fidgeting, can't sit still or remain seated, climbs/runs excessively, blurts out answers, can't wait for turn, interrupts, easily distracted

- **Oppositional Defiant Disorder**
  - Symptoms: angry and irritable mood, argumentative and defiant behavior, or vindictiveness

- **Anxiety Disorders**
  - Symptoms: excessive worrying, nervousness, shyness, avoiding places and activities, fear of objects or situations, panic attacks, separation anxiety

Slide 19

Symptoms of Psychosis

- **Pressure to keep talking**
- **Talks in mixed or garbled way**
- **Paranoid delusions**
- **Grandiose delusions**
- **Delusions of doom & disaster**
- **Skin picking and self harm**
- **Talking to self**
- **Bizarre behavior**

Slide 20

How it all comes together in treatment!

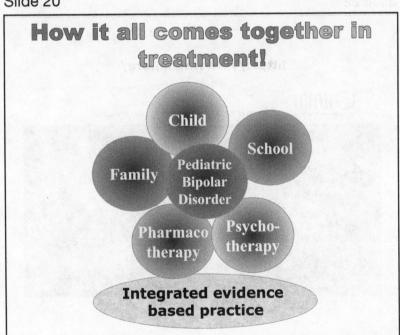

Child

School

Family

Pediatric Bipolar Disorder

Pharmaco therapy

Psycho-therapy

Integrated evidence based practice

Slide 21

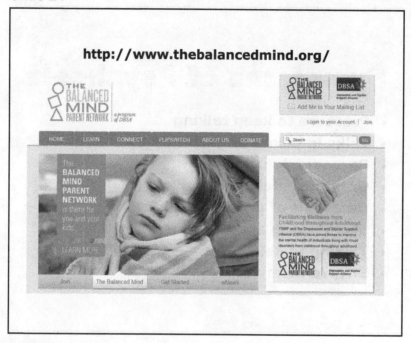

Slide 22

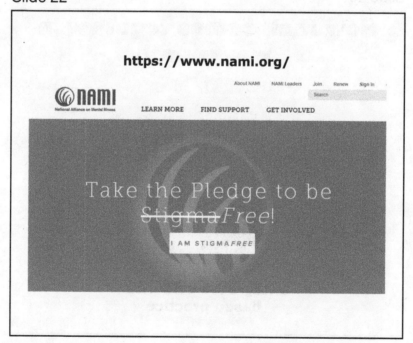

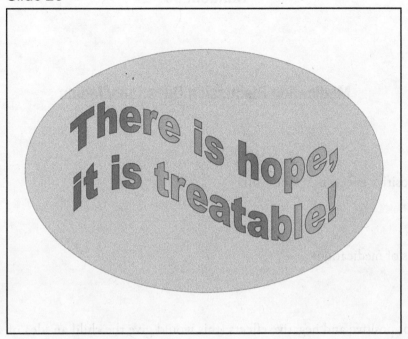

Handout #8

Medication Discussion Questions/Topics

1) Benefits/positive effects of medications

2) Side effects of medications

3) Timeline of positive and negative effects (this would give the child an idea of what to expect and to not be discouraged if the bad side effects come first)

4) Feeling different because of having to take medication

5) How much was the child told (i.e., psychoeducation) about meds up front—would more information have helped the child adjust to the process?

6) Are there things that the child specifically thinks that other children should know when starting/taking meds for bipolar disorder?

7) Tips for medication compliance

8) How do parents and doctors help?

Daily Mood Calendar

Name: _____   **Month:** _____

> Color in the square using a color that best described your overall mood for each part of the day.
>
> **KEY:**
> Blue = Sad
> Red = Angry/Explosive
> Gray = Crabby/Irritable
> Yellow = Happy
> Orange = Silly
> Green = Neutral/Fair
> Purple = Worried

Week 1   **Date** _____ **To** _____

	Sunday	Monday	Tuesday	Wednesday	Thursday	Friday	Saturday
Morning							
Afternoon							
Evening							

Week 2   **Date** _____ **To** _____

	Sunday	Monday	Tuesday	Wednesday	Thursday	Friday	Saturday
Morning							
Afternoon							
Evening							

Try at Home!

Session 2

Caregivers:

✓ Finding a way to talk about your child's symptoms in a language that everyone understands can be very helpful. This week, try to identify *three symptoms* that your child exhibits. Talk with your child about these symptoms: Does your child notice the symptom? Do you call it the same thing? Come up with names for your child's signature symptoms that you can use at home, with your family, and in treatment (for example, "meltdown," "volcano," or even "Bob"!).

✓ Mood monitoring is an important part of treatment. It helps the child, the caregiver, and the therapist see patterns in the child's mood fluctuations, and also helps us identify the things that trigger these mood fluctuations. Complete your own Mood Calendar for your child during the week.

✓ Help your child fill out a Mood Calendar for the next two weeks. When you notice that your child is experiencing a particular emotion, help the child label that emotion using the Mood Calendar's Feelings Legend and have the child color in the feeling.

Child:

✓ Become a Feelings Expert! Fill out the Mood Calendar for the next two weeks. Do this by coloring in the square with a color that BEST MATCHES how you feel, three times a day, every day for the next two weeks.

Thanks and Have a Great Week!

Handout #11

Establishing Routines

Important Activities to Target in Our Family

1. _____
2. _____
3. _____
4. _____

Ways We Can Establish These Routines

1. _____
   _____
   _____

2. _____
   _____
   _____

3. _____
   _____
   _____

4. _____
   _____

How Will We Monitor These Routines???

_____
_____
_____
_____
_____

Try at Home!

Session 3

Caregivers:

✓ Predictable and simplified routines are very important for your child, and they may reduce your child's frustration and reactivity. This week, pick one or more important areas to target for establishing a simple, consistent routine (for example: bedtime; morning school preparation). Discuss this routine with your child and create reminders of the routine (for example: posted schedules on the refrigerator). Do your best to stick to the routine this week!

✓ Identifying our feelings is an important first step in dealing with those feelings. This week, try a few strategies to help your child learn to identify and name his or her feelings—for example, reading a book about feelings, helping your child name the emotion that he or she is experiencing, or helping your child fill out a "My feeling today is . . ." worksheet.

✓ Begin trying new ways of handling your child's anger. If an anger episode occurs this week, remember the idea of **"putting out the fire"** to remain calm and help de-escalate the situation.

Child:

✓ Keep filling out your Mood Calendar. Do this by coloring in the square with a color that BEST MATCHES how you feel, three times a day, every day for the next week.

Thanks and Have a Great Week!

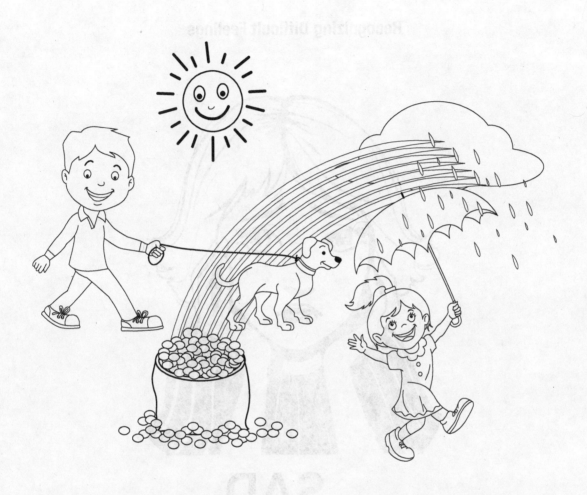

Recognizing Difficult Feelings

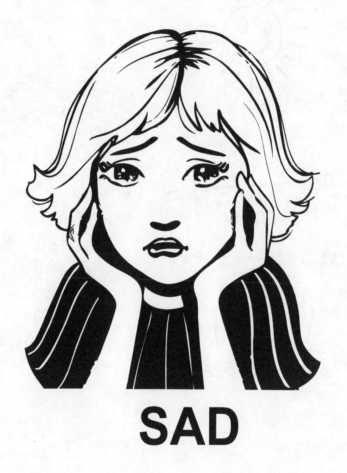

SAD

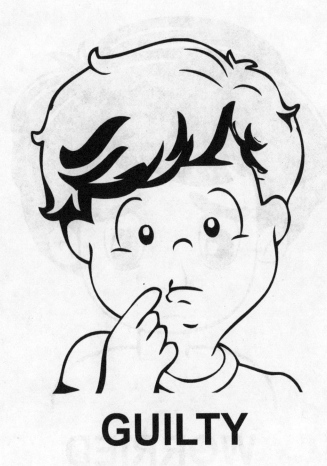

GUILTY

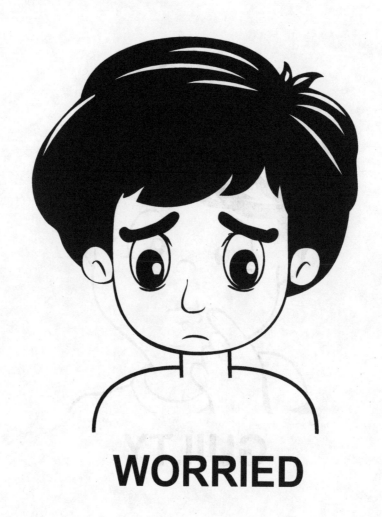

WORRIED

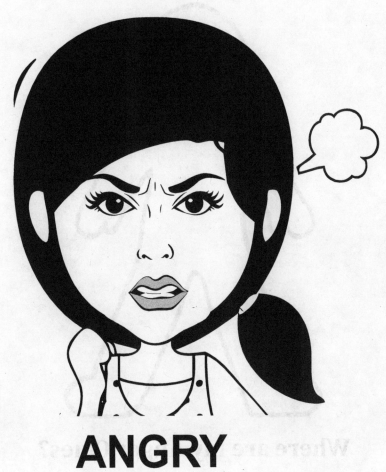

ANGRY

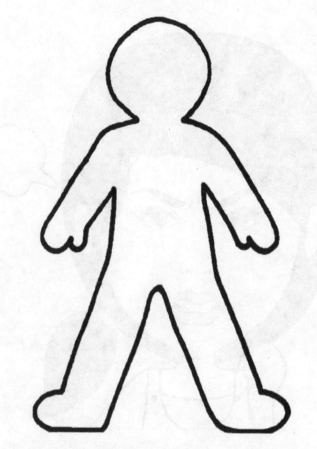

Where are my Anger Clues?

<u>Feelings</u> are something you <u>feel</u> in your <u>body</u>!

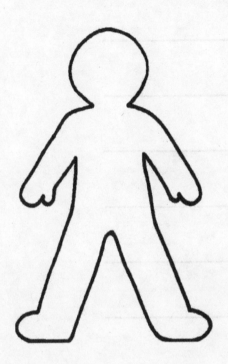

Color the places <u>YOU</u> feel your feelings...

<u>KEY:</u>

Blue = Sad

Red = Angry/Explosive

Gray = Crabby/Irritable

Yellow = Happy

Orange = Silly

Green = Neutral/Fair

Purple = Worried

What Are My Bugs???

1) _____

2) _____

3) _____

4) _____

5) _____

6) _____

7) _____

8) _____

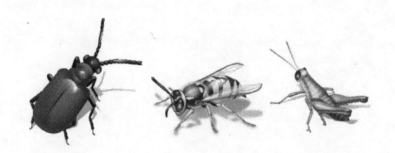

Handout #18

Session 4 Highlights for Parents and Caregivers

<u>A</u>ffect Regulation

During my session today, my therapist and I are going to:

✓ Look over my Mood Calendar to see if there are any *patterns* to my moods. This is important because then we can learn ways to increase my good feelings and decrease my difficult feelings (like *mad, cranky,* or *sad*). Also, doing my Mood Calendar can help me be more aware of how I'm feeling in the moment so I can express my feelings, and maybe even do something to help my difficult feelings.

✓ Talk about difficult feelings I've had before (like *sad, angry, nervous, guilty*), and what might have caused those feelings. Everyone has difficult feelings, and there is nothing wrong with having them. But I can do things to help myself, like say how I'm feeling and express my feelings without hurting myself or others.

✓ Talk about my ANGER CLUES. When I feel angry, it's kind of like a volcano: my anger bubbles up inside just like lava bubbles up in a volcano, and sometimes I may "explode" out of control. But there are *CLUES* in my body that tell me when I'm getting angry. This is my warning that the lava is bubbling up and something better be done before my anger volcano explodes. Be sure to ask me or my therapist what my *Anger Clues* are!

✓ Talk about the situations where I feel angry and experience my *Anger Clues*. These situations bug me, and so we call them my *bugs*. Soon I will start learning things to do to deal with my bugs.

How you can help me this week:

✓ Help me express my feelings, and help me put those feelings on my Mood Calendar. Are there any patterns to my moods?

✓ Help me recognize my Anger Clues if you notice them.

Things That Make Me Feel Good

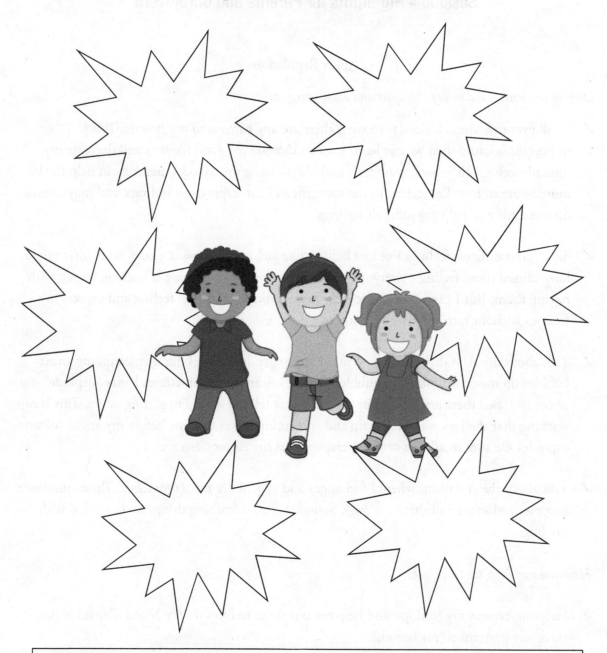

Write down or draw the places, activities, or people that make you feel good.

Handout #20

Nice Thoughts About Myself

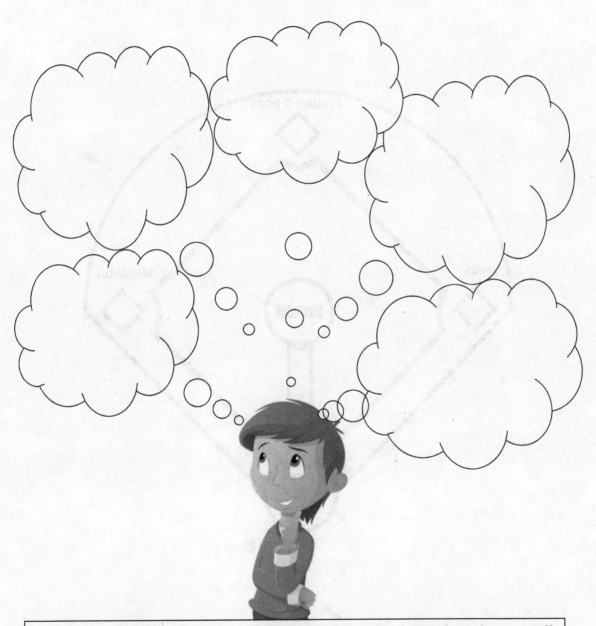

Fill in the thought bubbles by writing or drawing the nice thoughts that you have about yourself.

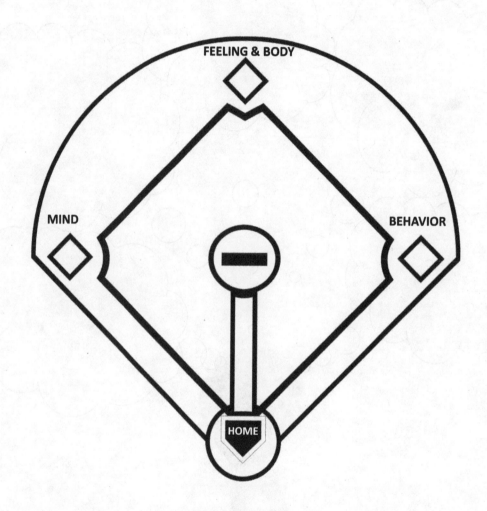

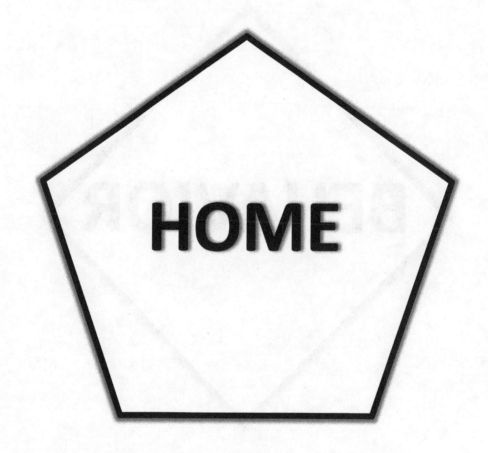

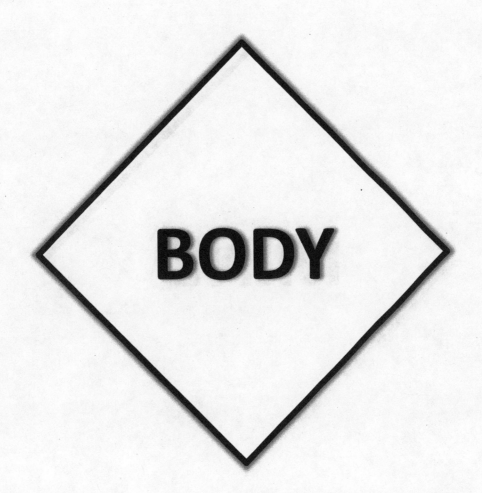

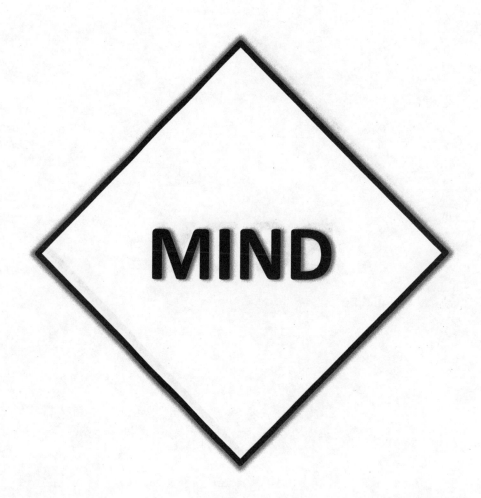

What can I **THINK** to feel better?

My BUG:

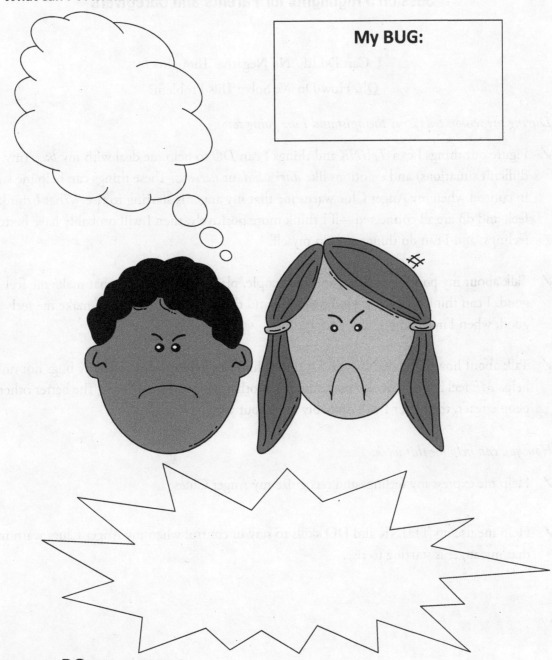

What can I **DO** To Feel Better?

Handout #23

Session 5 Highlights for Parents and Caregivers

I Can Do It! / **N**o **N**egative Thoughts /
Oh, How Do We Solve This Problem?

During my session today, my therapist and I are going to:

✓ Figure out things I can *THINK* and things I can *DO* to help me deal with my *bugs* (my difficult situations) and emotions like *angry, sad*, or *nervous*. These things can help me stay in control when my Anger Clue warns me that my anger is starting to rise. What I think, feel, and do are all connected—if I think more positively, then I will probably have better feelings, and I can do things to help myself.

✓ Talk about my positive qualities and the people, places, and activities that make me feel good. I can think about my good qualities, and the things or people that make me feel good, when I'm feeling upset or angry.

✓ Talk about how THINKING and DOING things to help me deal with my bugs not only helps *ME* feel better, but also may affect how other people react *TO me*. The better other people react, the better I will probably feel about yself.

How you can help me this week:

✓ Help me express my feelings and recognize my Anger Clues.

✓ Help me use my THINK and DO skills to stay in control when my Anger Clues warn me that my anger is starting to rise.

Handout #24

My Child's Competencies

1. _____

2. _____

3. _____

4. _____

5. _____

6. _____

7. _____

8. _____

9. _____

10. _____

Handout #25

Resources on Mindful Parenting

Websites

- 12 Exercises for Mindful Parenting: http://www.hillcrestschool.ca/media/files/12%20 Exercises%20for%20Mindful%20Parenting%202.pdf
- Mindful Parenting Resources from the Child Mind Institute: http://childmind.org/article/ mindful-parenting/
- Discussion Guide: http://mindfullifetoday.com/wp-content/uploads/Mindful-Parenting- Discussion-Guide-201508.pdf

Books

- Kabat-Zinn, M., & Kabat-Zinn, J. (1998). *Everyday Blessings: The Inner Work of Mindful Parenting*. New York: Hachette Books.
- Race, K. (2014). *Mindful Parenting: Simple and Powerful Solutions for Raising Creative, Engaged, Happy Kids in Today's Hectic World*. New York: St. Martin's Griffin.

Handout #26

Watching Thoughts Drift By: Instructions

1. First, I would like to ask your permission to do another mindfulness exercise. Are you willing to go ahead with that? [Get clients' permission and then move on.]

2. Just get in a comfortable position in your chair. Sit upright with your feet flat on the floor, your arms and legs uncrossed, and your hands resting in your lap, palms up or down, whichever is more comfortable. Allow your eyes to close gently [pause 10 seconds].

3. Take a few moments to get in touch with the physical sensations in your body, especially the sensations of touch or pressure where your body makes contact with the chair or floor [pause 10 seconds].

4. It is okay for your mind to wander away to thoughts, worries, images, bodily sensations, or feelings. Notice these thoughts and feelings and acknowledge their presence. Just observe passively the flow of your thoughts, one after another, without trying to figure out their meaning or their relationship to one another. As best you can, bring an attitude of allowing and gentle acceptance to your experience. There is nothing to be "fixed." Simply allow your experience to be your experience, without needing it to be other than what it is [pause 15 seconds].

5. Now, please imagine sitting next to a stream [pause 10 seconds]. As you gaze at the stream, you notice a number of leaves on the surface of the water. Keep looking at the leaves and watch them slowly drift downstream from left to right [pause 15 seconds].

6. Now, when thoughts come along into your mind, put each one on a leaf, and observe as each leaf comes closer to you. Then watch it slowly moving away from you, eventually drifting out of sight. Return to gazing at the stream, waiting for the next leaf to float by with a new thought [pause 10 seconds]. If one comes along, again, watch it come closer to you and then let it drift out of sight. Think whatever thoughts you think and allow them to flow freely on each leaf, one by one. Imagine your thoughts floating by like leaves down a stream [pause 15 seconds].

7. You can also allow yourself to take the perspective of the stream, just like in the chessboard exercise. Being the stream, you hold each of the leaves and notice the thought that each leaf carries as it sails by. You need not interfere with them—just let them flow and do what they do [pause 15 seconds].

8. Then, when you are ready, let go of those thoughts and gradually widen your attention to take in the sounds around you in this room [pause 10 seconds]. Take a moment to make the intention to bring this sense of gentle allowing and self-acceptance into the present moment . . . and when you are ready, slowly open your eyes.

Note: Republished with permission of New Harbinger Publications, from Eifert, G. H., & Forsyth, J. P. (2005), *Acceptance and Commitment Therapy for Anxiety Disorders: A Practitioner's Treatment Guide to Using Mindfulness, Acceptance, and Values-Based Behavior Change Strategies*. © Georg H. Eifert and John P. Forsyth/New Harbinger Publications, 2005. Permission conveyed through Copyright Clearance Center, Inc.

Handout #27

Try at Home!

Session 6

Caregivers:

✓ Many children with bipolar disorder often feel incompetent—much attention is given to their problematic emotions and behavior, and not to their *strengths*. You can help such children recognize their strengths (and build their self-esteem) by pointing out these strengths and giving equal attention to what they do well. This week, talk with your child about his or her strengths.

✓ You can also help raise your child's self-esteem by encouraging activities that build on these strengths—activities where your child can do *well*. If possible, figure out one or two activities your child can do that will promote his or her strengths (for example, doing an art project, taking a music or dance class, or enrolling in sports at a local park district).

✓ Talk with your child about **positive statements** she or he can say to her- or himself (giving a "pep talk"). Together, figure out some strengths that your child can remember to think of during the day. For times of difficulty, help your child come up with **coping "scripts"** he or she can use when feeling depressed or angry. This script may focus on the child's strengths, previous experiences where the child has dealt with the feeling successfully, calming thoughts, and so on. Typing the "script" on the computer, or making it an art project, may help make these stick.

✓ Time to focus on you! This week, practice using **mindfulness** techniques. Begin to incorporate mindfulness parenting strategies.

Thanks and Have a Great Week!

Feelings Charades

Print pages 2 and 3 double sided

SAD | MAD

SCARED | NERVOUS/
WORRIED

CRABBY | SILLY

Look, Act, Say

MAD

I know I'm mad if...
When mad, I can...

Look, Act, Say

SAD

I know I'm sad if...
When sad, I can...

Look, Act, Say

NERVOUS/ WORRIED

I know I'm nervous if...
When nervous, I can...

Look, Act, Say

SCARED

I know I'm scared if...
When scared, I can...

Look, Act, Say

SILLY

I know I'm silly if...
When silly, I can...

Look, Act, Say

CRABBY

I know I'm crabby if...
When crabby, I can...

Back straight

Eye contact

Mouth to speak clearly

Ears to listen

Handout #30

_____'s Definition of Respect:

_____

_____

_____

_____

_____

"I" MESSAGES

I FEEL . . .
(angry, sad, cranky, frustrated, worried . . .)

BECAUSE . . .
(reason why you feel that way)

AND I WOULD LIKE IF YOU . . .
(state what you would LIKE the other person to do to help the situation)

Session 7: Highlights for Parents and Caregivers

Be a Good Friend

During my session today, my therapist and I are going to talk about good communication skills like:

✓ Communicating my emotions nonverbally, and recognizing how other people may be feeling, based on the way they look and act: Even if I can't explain how I'm feeling, others may be able to tell how I'm feeling by the way I'm looking or acting. It's also helpful for me to figure out how other people may be feeling by how they look and act. We practiced ways people look and act when they have different feelings.

✓ Ways to express myself that show respect to myself and others: We practiced this by using "BEME" skills: Back straight; Eye Contact; Mouth to speak clearly; Ears to listen.

✓ Showing respect to others through my actions (like listening, paying attention, and not talking back), instead of showing disrespect: When I show respect, people react very differently than when I show disrespect.

✓ Using "I" messages to help other people understand *how* I feel and *why* I feel that way when I am bugged: "I" messages are like this: "I feel . . . because. . . ." This is very different from yelling and acting out of anger.

How you can help me this week:

✓ Remind me to use my *BEME* skills and *"I" messages*, especially when I am bugged!

✓ Help me express my feelings and recognize my Anger Clues, and remind me to mark down my feelings on my Mood Calendar.

✓ Play *Feelings Charades* with me to practice nonverbal expression of feelings.

Balanced Lifestyle

<u>**MY SELF-CARE NEEDS:**</u>

<u>**WAYS I CAN IMPROVE MY SELF-CARE THIS WEEK**</u> *(take time to eat breakfast, 10 minute walk, calling a friend, etc.)*

<u>**ENJOYABLE ACTIVITIES I WANT TO ADD INTO MY LIFE:**</u>

PIE CHART: CURRENT life activities (% time spent in work, child care, housework, etc. AND positive experiences, social activities, relaxation, etc.)	**CREATING BALANCE:** Redistribute the percentages to carve out time for self-care and create balance in your life.

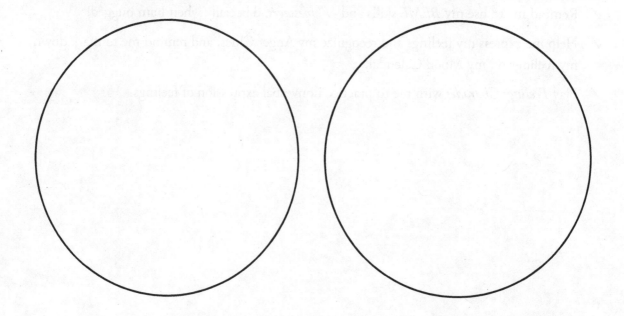

Handout #34

Try at Home!

Session 8

Caregivers:

✓ Positive friendships can go a long way in helping your child. You can help your child make and keep friends by setting up play dates, sleepovers, or supervised group activities. This week, talk with your child about setting up a structured activity with other kids.

✓ Tough situations (your child's *bugs*) are going to happen. But these can be prevented or prepared for to lessen the amount of distress your child feels. Set aside time this week, when everyone is calm, to talk with your child about their "bugs." Help your child feel understood by sharing your own thoughts and feelings (remember to use "I" messages!) As a team, practice ways your child can express their emotions and use their THINK and DO skills to prevent the anger from exploding.

✓ But sometimes the anger still explodes. If emotional outbursts occur this week, practice ways to "put out the fire"—remain calm, help your child soothe themselves, remove your child from the distressing situation and take them to a safe zone, and make sure everyone is safe.

✓ Remember that timing is KEY! After the fire has been put out, come up with appropriate consequences for the episode. Also, talk with your child about what everyone can do next time to handle the situation.

✓ Time to focus on you! It's so important to recharge our own batteries. Begin to incorporate self-care activities in your own life to create greater balance.

Thanks and Have a Great Week!

Handout #35

Try at Home!

Session 9

✓ As family, create a plan for dealing with difficult situations. What THINK and DO skills can everyone use to deal with **triggers** or **"bugs"**? Practice these this week and pick the best responses.

✓ Also create a family plan for dealing with **rage episodes** once they occur. For example, caregivers can remain calm and remove their child from the distressing interaction; siblings can move to another room and begin an enjoyable activity; and so on. Again, practice many different options, and choose the most helpful response.

✓ Remember to pay attention to the positive experiences, too! Praise your children when they help each other, get along well, or use the family coping plans.

Thanks and Have a Great Week!

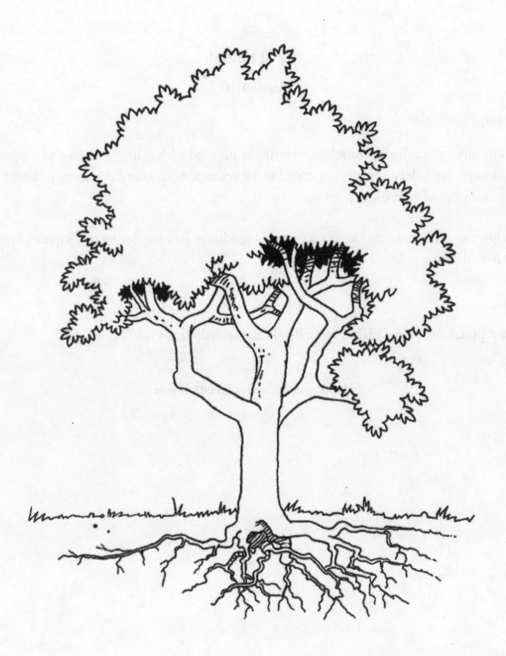

Try at Home!

Session 10

Caregivers:

✓ A huge part of caring for ourselves is staying connected with others who give us support. This week, try at least one new or added social activity. Also, take the time to talk with a core member of your support group.

✓ Help your child make and keep supportive friendships by completing the Support Tree activity together at home.

Child:

✓ Keep practicing your THINK and DO skills! Get help from your family, too.

Thanks and Have a Great Week!

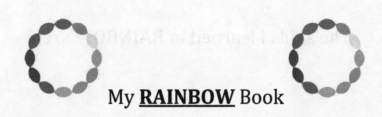

My **RAINBOW** Book

My name is

I am   years old

My therapist's name is

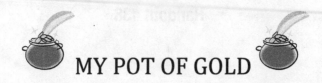

MY POT OF GOLD

The skills I learned in RAINBOW are...

FAVORITE **RAINBOW** ACTIVITY

My favorite parts of RAINBOW were...

RAINBOW & MY FAMILY

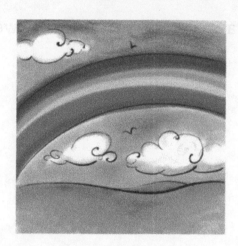

Some things that are better in our family since we started coming to RAINBOW ...

Amy E. West is an associate professor of clinical psychology in psychiatry and a licensed clinical psychologist in the Pediatric Mood Disorders Program in the Department of Psychiatry at the University of Illinois at Chicago. Her research broadly focuses on the use of psychosocial interventions in the treatment of pediatric mood disorders. She was funded by the National Institutes of Mental Health to develop and study child- and family-focused cognitive-behavioral therapy, or CFF-CBT (the RAINBOW program), for children with bipolar spectrum disorders. Dr. West also has research interests in the developmental psychopathology of mood disorders in children, treatment mechanisms in psychosocial interventions, suicidal behavior in pediatric bipolar disorder, and developing psychosocial treatments that are culturally relevant to unique populations. Dr. West received a Bachelor of Arts degree in psychology from Stanford University and her doctorate in clinical psychology from the University of Virginia, and she completed her pre-doctoral internship and post-doctoral fellowship in child/pediatric psychology at Harvard Medical School/Children's Hospital in Boston.

Sally M. Weinstein is an assistant professor of clinical psychology in psychiatry and a licensed clinical psychologist in the Pediatric Mood Disorders Program in the Department of Psychiatry at the University of Illinois at Chicago. She is engaged in programs of research investigating the psychosocial treatment of children with bipolar disorder, and the assessment and treatment of suicidality within pediatric bipolar disorder. Dr. Weinstein also provides clinical evaluations and treatment for children and adolescents with mood disorders and facilitates the CFF-CBT/RAINBOW group therapy program for children with bipolar disorder. Dr. Weinstein received a Bachelor of Science degree from Duke University and obtained her doctorate in clinical psychology from the University of Illinois at Chicago. Dr. Weinstein completed her internship in child clinical and pediatric psychology at La Rabida Children's Hospital in Chicago, Illinois, and completed a two-year postdoctoral fellowship, funded by the National Institutes of Health, within the Pediatric Mood Disorders Program at the University of Illinois at Chicago.

Mani N. Pavuluri is board-certified in general and child and adolescent psychiatry; a Distinguished Fellow of the American Academy of Child and Adolescent Psychiatry; Fellow of the American College of Neuropsychopharmacology; professor, and the founding director of the Pediatric Mood Disorders Program, Department of Psychiatry, University of Illinois at Chicago. She completed adult and child psychiatry training through the Royal Australian and New Zealand College of Psychiatrists and at the Rush Presbyterian Medical Center in Chicago. She had been funded by the National Institutes of Health and private foundations to study brain function in bipolar disorder. She serves on several editorial boards of international scientific journals.